CBS Confident Pharmacy Series

Pharmacology

Course Code: ER20-21T

for **Second Year Diploma in Pharmacy**

As per latest syllabus prescribed by Pharmacy Council of India

Salient Features

- Lucid and easy language
- To the point answers
- Remembering the concepts in the simplest way
- Infusing confidence in the reader to appear in the board examinations

Other books by the same author under

CBS Confident Pharmacy Series

- *Social Pharmacy* for First Year Diploma in Pharmacy
- *Pharmaceutics, 4/e* for First Year Diploma in Pharmacy
- *Pharmacognosy, 4/e* for First Year Diploma in Pharmacy
- *Pharmaceutical Chemistry, 4/e* for First Year Diploma in Pharmacy
- *Human Anatomy and Physiology, 4/e* for First Year Diploma in Pharmacy
- *Pharmacy Law and Ethics* for Second Year Diploma in Pharmacy
- *Biochemistry and Clinical Pathology, 4/e* for Second Year Diploma in Pharmacy
- *Hospital and Clinical Pharmacy, 4/e* for Second Year Diploma in Pharmacy
- *Pharmacotherapeutics* for Second Year Diploma in Pharmacy
- *Community Pharmacy and Management* for Second Year Diploma in Pharmacy

CBS Confident Pharmacy Series

Pharmacology

Course Code: ER20-21T

for **Second Year Diploma in Pharmacy**

As per latest syllabus prescribed by Pharmacy Council of India

VN Raje MPharm, MBA

Principal
Gourishankar Education Society's
GES College of Pharmacy (DPharm)
Limb, Satara, Maharashtra

CBSPD

CBS Publishers & Distributors Pvt Ltd

New Delhi • Bengaluru • Chennai • Kochi • Kolkata • Lucknow • Mumbai
Hyderabad • Jharkhand • Nagpur • Patna • Pune • Uttarakhand

CBS Confident Pharmacy Series

Pharmacology

Course Code: ER20-21T
for **Second Year Diploma in Pharmacy**

As per latest syllabus prescribed by Pharmacy Council of India

Disclaimer

Science and technology are constantly changing fields. New research and experience broaden the scope of information and knowledge. The author has tried his best in giving information available to him while preparing the material for this book. Although, all efforts have been made to ensure optimum accuracy of the material, yet it is quite possible some errors might have been left uncorrected. The publisher, the printer and the author will not be held responsible for any inadvertent errors or inaccuracies.

ISBN: 978-93-5466-502-8

First Edition: 2023
Reprint: 2024 2025

Published by Satish Kumar Jain and produced by Varun Jain for

CBS Publishers & Distributors Pvt Ltd
4819/XI Prahlad Street, 24 Ansari Road, Daryaganj, New Delhi 110 002, India
Ph: 011-23289259, 23266861 Website: www.cbspd.com
e-mail: delhi@cbspd.com

Corporate Office: 204 FIE, Industrial Area, Patparganj, Delhi 110 092
Ph: 011-4934 4934 Fax: 011-4934 4935 e-mail: publishing@cbspd.com; publicity@cbspd.com

Branches

- **Bengaluru:** Seema House 2975, 17th Cross, KR Road, Banasankari 2nd Stage, Bengaluru 560 070, Karnataka, India
  Ph: +91-80-26771678/79 Fax: +91-80-26771680 e-mail: bangalore@cbspd.com
- **Chennai:** 7, Subbaraya Street, Shenoy Nagar, Chennai 600 030, Tamil Nadu, India
  Ph: +91-44-26680620, 26681266 Fax: +91-44-42032115 e-mail: chennai@cbspd.com
- **Kochi:** 42/1325, 1326, Power House Road, Opp KSEB, Power House, Ernakulam, Kochi 682 018, India
  Ph: +91-484-4059061–65 Fax: +91-484-4059065 e-mail: kochi@cbspd.com
- **Kolkata:** 147, Hind Ceramics Compound, 1st Floor, Nilgunj Road, Belghoria, Kolkata 700 056, West Bengal, India
  Ph: +91-33-25633055–56 e-mail: kolkata@cbspd.com
- **Lucknow:** Basement, Khushnuma Complex, 7-Meerabai Marg (behind Jawahar Bhawan), Lucknow 226 001, India
  Ph: +91-522-4000032 e-mail: tiwari.lucknow@cbspd.com
- **Mumbai:** PWD Shed. Gala no. 25/26, Ramchandra Bhatt Marg, Next to JJ Hospital Gate no. 2, Opp. Union Bank of India, Noorbaug Mumbai 400 009, Maharashtra, India
  Ph: +91-22-66661880/89 e-mail: mumbai@cbspd.com

Representatives

- **Hyderabad** 0-9885175004 • **Jharkhand** 0-9811541605 • **Nagpur** 0-9421945513
- **Patna** 0-9334159340 • **Pune** 0-9923910676 • **Uttarakhand** 0-9716462459

Printed at Mudrak, Noida, UP, India

Preface

This book **Pharmacology** under the CBS Confident Pharmacy Series which builds self-confidence in students which helps to get success in the examinations. The book has been written to meet the requirements of students of Diploma in Pharmacy (D Pharm) in accordance with the new revised syllabus ER2020 prescribed by Pharmacy Council of India.

This book is small and humble effort has been put in for compiling necessary information on the subject. An attempt has been made to demystify and simplify the basic concepts for the students of pharmacy and to enable them get an evergreen success in MSBTE examinations and all other qualifying examinations throughout India.

The salient features of the present book are:

- Lucid and easy language
- To the point answers
- Remembering facts in the simplest way
- Infusing confidence in the reader to appear in the board examinations.

Hence, the series is named

CBS Confident Pharmacy Series

I am confident that this book will be useful to both the students and the teachers of Diploma in Pharmacy as well as the candidates desiring to succeed in competitive examinations for better job opportunities in pharmacy profession such as hospital pharmacists in PHCs, civil hospitals, etc.

Vijay N Raje

to

my beloved family

Acknowledgements

I express my heartfelt thanks to Prof Madan Jagtap, Chairman, Gourishankar Education Society, Satara, Maharashtra, for consistent encouragement and inspiration for writing this book.

I wish to acknowledge the prompt and efficient help given by Prof Milind Jagtap, Mr Jaywant Salunkhe, Mr Appa Rajage, Mr Nitin Mudalgikar, and Mr Shrirang Katekar of Gourishankar Education Society, Satara.

I am also thankful to Shri Satish Kumar Jain, Chairman and Managing Director, and Shri Shantanu Sarkar, Assistant General Manager, Mumbai Branch, CBS Publishers & Distributors Pvt Ltd, for their sustained efforts and keen interest in the publication of this book.

I wish all my beloved students to have a great success in the board examinations.

Vijay N Raje

Syllabus

(As per PCI New ER 2020)

Pharmacology

Course Code: ER20-21T

1. **General Pharmacology**
   - Introduction and scope of Pharmacology
   - Various routes of drug administration—advantages and disadvantages
   - Drug absorption—definition, types, factors affecting drug absorption
   - Bioavailability and the factors affecting bioavailability
   - Drug distribution—definition, factors affecting drug distribution
   - Biotransformation of drugs—definition, types of biotransformation reactions, factors influencing drug metabolisms
   - Excretion of drugs—definition, routes of drug excretion
   - General mechanisms of drug action and factors modifying drug action
2. **Drugs Acting on the Peripheral Nervous System**
   - Steps involved in neurohumoral transmission
   - Definition, classification, pharmacological actions, dose, indication and contraindications of
     - a. Cholinergic drugs
     - b. Anti-cholinergic drugs
     - c. Adrenergic drugs
     - d. Anti-adrenergic drugs
     - e. Neuromuscular blocking agents
     - f. Drugs used in myasthenia gravis
     - g. Local anaesthetic agents
     - h. Non-steroidal anti-inflammatory drugs (NSAIDs)
3. **Drugs Acting on the Eye**

   Definition, classification, pharmacological actions, dose, indications and contraindications of
   - Miotics
   - Mydriatics
   - Drugs used in Glaucoma
4. **Drugs Acting on the Central Nervous System**

   Definition, classification, pharmacological actions, dose, indications, and contraindications of
   - General anaesthetics
   - Hypnotics and sedatives
   - Anti-convulsant drugs
   - Anti-anxiety drugs
   - Anti-depressant drugs
   - Anti-psychotics
   - Nootropic agents
   - Centrally acting muscle relaxants
   - Opioid analgesics
5. **Drugs Acting on the Cardiovascular System**

   Definition, classification, pharmacological actions, dose, indications and contraindications of
   - Anti-hypertensive drugs
   - Anti-anginal drugs
   - Anti-arrhythmic drugs
   - Drugs used in atherosclerosis and
   - Congestive heart failure
   - Drug therapy for shock

6. **Drugs Acting on Blood and Blood Forming Organs**
Definition, classification, pharmacological actions, dose, indications and contraindications of
- Hematinic agents
- Anti-coagulants
- Anti-platelet agents
- Thrombolytic drugs

7. **Drugs Acting on Respiratory System**
Definition, classification, pharmacological actions, dose, indications and contraindications of
- Bronchodilators
- Expectorants
- Anti-tussive agents
- Mucolytic agents

8. **Drugs Acting on the Gastrointestinal Tract**
Definition, classification, pharmacological actions, dose, indications and contraindications of
- Anti-ulcer drugs
- Anti-emetics
- Laxatives and purgatives
- Anti-diarrhoeal drugs

9. **Drugs Acting on the Kidney**
Definition, classification, pharmacological actions, dose, indications and contraindications of
- Diuretics
- Anti-diuretics

10. **Hormones and Hormone Antagonists**
Physiological and pathological role and clinical uses of
- Thyroid hormones
- Anti-thyroid drugs
- Parathormone
- Calcitonin
- Vitamin D
- Insulin
- Oral hypoglycemic agents
- Estrogen
- Progesterone
- Oxytocin
- Corticosteroids

11. **Autocoids**
- Physiological role of histamine, 5-HT and prostaglandins
- Classification, clinical uses and adverse effects of antihistamines and 5-HT antagonists

12. **Chemotherapeutic Agents:** Introduction, basic principles of chemotherapy of infections, infestations and neoplastic diseases, classification, dose, indication and contraindications of drugs belonging to following classes:
- Penicillins
- Cephalosporins
- Aminoglycosides
- Fluoroquinolones
- Macrolides
- Tetracyclines
- Sulphonamides
- Anti-tubercular drugs
- Anti-fungal drugs
- Anti-viral drugs
- Anti-amoebic agents
- Anthelmintics
- Anti-malarial agents
- Anti-neoplastic agents

13. **Biologicals**
Definition, types and indications of biological agents with examples

Contents

Chapter 1

General Pharmacology

- Scope of pharmacology
- Absorption of drugs
- Distribution of drug in the body
- Excretion/disposition of drugs (elimination of drugs)
- Routes of administration of drugs
- Bioavailability
- Biotransformation/metabolism of drugs
- Factors modifying drug action

Q 1. Define pharmacology. Explain scope of pharmacology.

Pharmacology

Pharmacology is the science, which deals with the study of drugs and their actions on human body or animals.

Pharmacology has two branches:

1. **Clinical pharmacology:** It deals with the study of action or effects of drugs in human being.
2. **Experimental pharmacology:** It deals with the action or effects of a drug on experimental animals.

Scope of Pharmacology

1. The knowledge of pharmacology is needed for the purpose of regular screening and testing of new drugs to determine their therapeutic uses, harmful effects, safety and efficacy on humans and animals.
2. The pharmacology has made its position in the medical field and in medicines of greater importance.
3. The scope of pharmacology includes the cultivation of medicinal plants which serves as drugs, the synthesis of chemical compounds of medicinal use.
4. Pharmacy is the allied branch of pharmacology, which is concerned with the collection, preparation and standardization of drugs.
5. The various branches of pharmacology provides knowledge of drugs to the world especially to the persons of medical, paramedical and nursing field category.
6. The knowledge of pharmacological principles is essential for maintenance of optimal health of the humanity and animals.
7. The allied fields/branches/subdivisions of pharmacology are:
   a. **Pharmacy:** It deals with the science and art of analysing standardising, compounding and dispensing of drugs, so as to make them fit for administration.

b. **Pharmacognosy:** It is a branch of pharmacy which deals with identification of drugs based on the study of physical, chemical botanical and some aspects of biological properties.
c. **Pharmacodynamics:** It deals with the site and mode of action of drugs on living organisms.
d. **Pharmacokinetics:** It deals with the study of absorption, distribution, metabolism and excretion of drugs and their relationship to the pharmacological response.
e. **Pharmacotherapeutics:** It means various methods and systems that are used in prevention and treatment of diseases.
f. **Toxicology:** It is the science which deals with the adverse effects of the drugs and study of poisons.
g. **Posology:** It deals with the study of doses of the drugs.
h. **Chemotherapy:** It is defined as the use of chemical compounds in the treatment of infectious diseases so as to destroy the microorganisms without damaging host tissues.
i. **Clinical pharmacology:** It involves the principles of clinical drug evaluation that apply to medicine.
j. **Therapeutics:** It is a general term describing the use of drugs in the treatment of disease.
k. **Pharmacogenetics:** This area of pharmacology examines relation of genetic factors to variations in response to drugs.
l. **Pharmacoeconomics:** It deals with the study of the analysis of cost of drug therapy to the health care system and the society.
m. **Clinical pharmacy:** It involves co-operation of the pharmacist with the physician in educating the patient about compliance and counselling him on how to take the medication and monitoring the errors in taking the drugs.

Q 2. Define 'pharmacology'. Give the classification of drugs on the basis of source, nature and active constituent present in it.

Pharmacology

Pharmacology is defined as the study of effect of drugs on the living organism and its organs along with mechanism of action, adverse effects, and doses of the drugs.
The word pharmacology is derived from two Greek words, *pharmacon* → a drug, *logus* → to treat or science.

Classification of Drugs

a. As per Source of Drugs

1. Plants, e.g. morphine, digoxin, reserpine, vinblastin.
2. Animals, e.g. insulin, heparin, thyroid extract.

3. Minerals, e.g. liquid paraffin, magnesium sulphate, kaolin.
4. Synthetic, e.g. aspirin, sulphonamides, corticosteroids.
5. Microorganisms, e.g. penicillins, tetracyclines, rifampicin, cephalosporins, l-asparaginase.

b. As per Nature of Drugs

The drugs from plant origin contain pharmacologically active constituents such as:

1. Alkaloids, e.g. reserpine, morphine, emetine, atropine.
2. Glycosides, e.g. digoxin, strophanthin.
3. Oils:
   a. Fixed oils, e.g. olive oil, castor oil, cod-liver oil,
   b. Volatile oil, e.g. clove oil, eucalyptus oil, turpentine oil.
4. Resins, e.g. podophyllum resin.
5. Gums, e.g. agar, acacia, tragacanth.
6. Tannins, e.g. catechu, tannic acid.
7. Hormones, e.g. insulin, sex hormones.

Q 3. Give the classification of routes of administration of drugs.

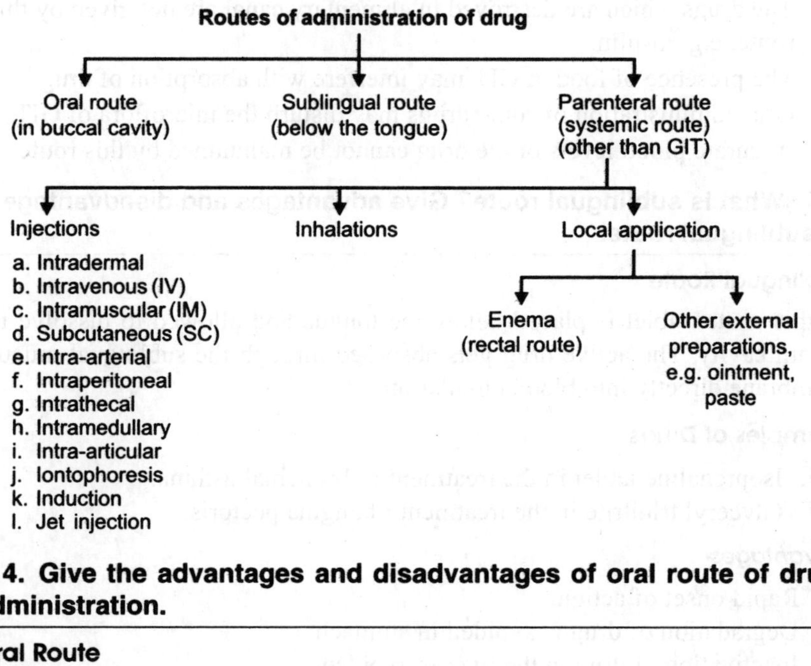

Q 4. Give the advantages and disadvantages of oral route of drug administration.

Oral Route

In this route, the drug is placed in oral cavity and is swallowed along with water or milk, etc.

Advantages

1. It is a common and safe route of drug administration.
2. No special skill is required for administration of drug.
3. It is very convenient route.
4. Sterilisation is not required for the preparations taken orally.
5. There are low possibilities of adverse reactions.
6. This route is applicable from infants up to aged patients.
7. The large quantity of drug can be administered by this route.
8. Preparations like syrup, mixture, tablet, capsule, pills are administered by this route.

Disadvantages

1. Onset of action is slow.
2. Absorption of certain drugs is irregular and negligible.
3. This route is not useful in clinical emergencies.
4. The irritant and unpalatable drugs cannot be administered by this route.
5. This route is not useful in cases of unconscious and incooperative patients.
6. This route is not useful in prevomiting and diarrhoea patients.
7. The drugs which are destroyed in alimentary canal are not given by this route, e.g. insulin.
8. The presence of food in GIT may interfere with absorption of drug.
9. Oral administration of some drugs may disturb the microflora of GIT.
10. Accurate blood levels of the drug cannot be maintained by this route.

Q 5. What is sublingual route? Give advantages and disadvantages of sublingual route.

Sublingual Route

In this route, tablet is placed below the tongue and allowed to dissolve in mouth cavity. The active drug gets absorbed through the sublingual mucus membrane directly into blood circulation.

Examples of Drugs

i. Isoprenaline tablet in the treatment of bronchial asthma.
ii. Glyceryl trinitrite in the treatment of angina pectoris.

Advantages

1. Rapid onset of action.
2. Degradation of drug is avoided in stomach.
3. Inactivation of drug in the liver is avoided.
4. If tablet is found to be toxic, it can be spit out easily.
5. Presence of food in GIT does not affect the absorption of drug.

Disadvantages

1. Not suitable for large doses and frequent use of drug.
2. Some drugs may cause irritation to buccal mucosa.
3. Excessive salivation may cause swallowing of drug.
4. The drugs having direct or toxic effects should be administered carefully to avoid side effects on heart.

Q 6. What is parenteral route? Give advantages and disadvantages of parenteral route.

Parenteral Route

The routes of administration of drug other than alimentary canal are called parenteral routes.

- In this case, the drug in the form of solution or suspension is injected in the body with the help of hollow needle and syringe.
- In some cases, drugs in the form of vapour or fine droplets are inhaled in respiratory tract or sometimes pastes are rubbed over the skin.

Advantages

1. Rapid onset of action.
2. The drugs which irritate the GIT, can be given by this route.
3. Accurate dose and accurate blood level of drug can be possible.
4. This route is useful in cases of vomiting and diarrhoea.
5. This route is useful in unconscious and uncooperative patients.
6. The drugs which are destroyed in GIT can be given by this route.
7. The smaller quantity of drugs is required by this route.
8. This route is useful in clinical emergencies.
9. The large quantities of drug are also administered by this route, e.g. saline solution.
10. 100% bioavailability is possible by IV route.

Disadvantages

1. This route is inconvenient to the patient and for frequent administration of drugs.
2. Skilled person is necessary for administration of drugs.
3. Strict aseptic technique is to be followed during drug administration.
4. The possibility of pain and edema at the site of application.
5. Self-medication is difficult.
6. The sterilization of syringe and needle is necessary.
7. The possibility of nerve damage.
8. Once the drug is absorbed in blood circulation, the adverse effects cannot be reversed or controlled.

Q 7. Explain various types of parenteral routes. Give their advantages and disadvantages.

a. Intradermal Route

In this route, the drug is injected in the dermis layer of the skin. Only a small quantity of drug can be administered by this route and the injection is painful.

Importance

i. This route is used for the detection of drug allergy, e.g. penicillin is injected intradermally to observe allergic reactions to it.
ii. Vaccines such as BCG, smallpox are administered by this route.

b. Intramuscular Route

In this route, drug is administered directly into the muscular tissue.

Advantages

1. Mild irritants, suspensions, colloids and injections with insoluble oily bases can be administered by this route.
2. The absorption of water-soluble drugs is rapid than subcutaneous or oral route.
3. Massaging and application of heat at the site of injection by IM route may increase the drug absorption.
4. The drugs administered by this route form tissue depots from where drug is slowly released and this provides prolonged duration of action.

Disadvantages

1. Sterilization of syringe and needle is essential.
2. Skilled person is required for drug administration.
3. Some drugs may cause tissue irritation and pains by intramuscular route.
4. If proper care is not taken there is an injury to the nerves.
5. Total volume of drug injected by IM route is restricted up to 10 ml.
6. Certain intramuscular injections require more time for absorption as compared to oral route.

c. Inhalation Route

In this route, the drug in the form of gas or in vapour form can be inhaled, e.g.

i. Isoprenaline spray is used in bronchial asthma.
ii. Volatile general anaesthetics are also given by this route.

Advantages

1. The absorption of drug by this route is very rapid.
2. The drug given by this route produces local as well as systemic effects.
3. Blood levels of volatile substances such as general anaesthetics can be conveniently controlled.

Disadvantages

1. The drug directly enters the left side of the heart, hence there is a danger of cardiac toxicity.
2. Certain drugs produce local irritation, may increase respiratory secretions.
3. Special apparatus such as automizer or nebuliser is needed for administration of drug.

d. Intravenous Route (IV Route)

In this route, the drug is injected directly into the lumen of vein. The drug produces rapid action and desired blood concentration can be achieved by a definite dose of a drug.

Advantages

1. The onset of drug action is very rapid.
2. This route is effective in clinical emergencies.
3. 100% absorption of drug is possible by this route.
4. Large quantity of drug can be administered by this route, e.g. normal saline solution.
5. The drug which produces irritation and pains by IM route can be given by this route.
6. The hypertonic solutions can be administered intravenously because the drug is diluted by bloodstream.
7. The accurate blood concentration of drug can be achieved by this route.
8. Only minimum quantity of drug is required to get a particular effect as compared to other routes.
9. Adjustment of additional dose and control on the rate of administration is possible by IV route.
10. Complete bioavailability of drug can be assured by IV route.

Disadvantages

1. Self-medication is difficult.
2. Sometimes, leakage of drug outside the vein produces severe irritation and abscess formation.
3. Sterilization of needle and syringe is essential.
4. Skilled person is essential for drug administration.
5. Speed of drug entering through IV set should be slow and constant supervision is necessary.
6. Once the drug is absorbed in the systemic circulation, the adverse effects of drug cannot be reversed or controlled.

e. Intra-arterial Route

- In this route the drug is administered directly into the artery.

- The drug produces a sudden high concentration in arterial blood and hence may be harmful locally or damaging to tissues supplied by the artery.
- This route has no advantages except in diagnostic studies, such as angiograms and in embolization therapy.
- Certain anti-malignancy compounds are administered by regional intra-arterial perfusing in localized malignancies.

f. Intraperitoneal Route

- This route has been sometimes used in infants for giving fluids like glucose, saline, as the peritoneum offers a large surface for absorption.
- This route is also used for peritoneal dialysis.

g. Intrathecal Route

- In this route involves introduction of drugs such as spinal anaesthetics into the subarachnoid space.
- The drugs act directly on the central nervous system.
- This route is also convenient for producing high local concentrations in the subarachnoid space.
- Examples:
  1. Certain antibiotics and antimalignancy drugs are given by this route.
  2. Lignocaine is now used extradurally to produce anaesthesia for pelvic surgery.

h. Intramedullary Route

It involves the introduction of a drug into the bone marrow and is now rarely used.

i. Intra-articular Route

- In this case the drugs are administered directly into a joint for treatment of local conditions.
- This ensures a high local concentration of the drug, e.g. hydrocortisone acetate in the treatment of rheumatoid arthritis.

j. Iontophoresis

- In this procedure, galvanic current is used for bringing about the penetration of drugs into the deeper tissues where they may act upon the tissues in the neighbourhood of the point of application.
- Anode iontophoresis is used for compounds bearing positive charge and cathode iontophoresis for the negatively charged compounds.
- The force of repulsion between similar charges drives the drug into the deeper tissues. salicylates have been used by this method.

k. Inuction

- Certain drugs when rubbed into the skin (inuction) can get absorbed and produces systemic effects.
- For example: Nitroglycerin ointment in angina pectoris.

l. Jet Injection (Dermojet)

- This method involves the transcutaneous introduction of a drug by means of a high velocity jet produced through a micro-fine orifice.
- This method does not require the use of a needle and is therefore painless.

m. Subcutaneous (SC) Route

In this route the drug is injected into the subcutaneous tissues of the thigh, abdomen and arm, e.g. adrenaline, insulin, etc.

Advantages of SC route	*Disadvantages of SC route*
• Actions of the drugs are sustained and uniform • Useful in diarrhoea and vomiting patients • Useful in unconscious patient • First pass effect is avoided • Self-medication is possible (e.g. insulin) • Depot preparations can be inserted	• Only non-irritant drugs can be given • Absorption of drug is slow than IM route • Expensive • Sterilization technique must be followed • Large volume of drug cannot be administered

Q 8. What is local/topical route? Give its advantages and disadvantages.

Local Route/Local Application/Topical Route

- In this route, the drugs are applied or administered to the localized or specific areas of the body.
- These preparations are to be meant for their action at the site of application, e.g. paste, ointment, drops, lotions.

Advantages

1. This route provides an easy administration of drug.
2. Local application is useful when prolonged effect of drug is required.
3. There is a low possibility of systemic absorption of the medicament.
4. No special skill or apparatus is required for administration.

Disadvantages

1. The drugs in the form of watery solution are sometimes absorbed into the blood and may produce undesirable effects.
2. The drugs like eyedrops may penetrate into the anterior chamber and affect ciliary muscles, e.g. cocaine.
3. Some drugs may show toxic effect at the site of application.

Q 9. What is rectal route of drug administration? Give its advantages and disadvantages. OR Write a note on 'rectal route'.

Rectal Route

The route of administration in which the drug in the form of solution is introduced into the rectum is called rectal route, e.g. enema preparation, suppository.

Advantages

1. When the drug produces irritation by oral route, this route may be used.
2. When patient does not swallow the drug, this route is preferred.
3. The children who do not cooperate in taking medicines by oral route, the rectal route may be recommended.
4. This route is used when local effects in the rectum are required.

Disadvantages

1. The absorption of drug is not complete because less surface area is available for absorption as compared to oral route.
2. This route is not liked by the patients.
3. A few drugs may produce local irritation of nasal mucosa.
4. Possibility of absorption of drug into blood and drug may be metabolized in the liver before reaching the target organ.

Q 10. Define the terms.

- **Agonist:** A drug which combines with receptor and gives a pharmacological response is called agonist.
- **Antagonist:** A drug which combines with receptor but does not produce pharmacological action and only blocks the receptor is called antagonist.
- **Affinity:** The ability of a drug to get bound to the receptor is called affinity of a drug for the receptor.
- **Efficacy or intrinsic activity:** The ability of a drug to give a pharmacological action after combination with receptor is called efficacy of a drug.
- **Receptor:** A receptor is a specific functional cellular component which when combines with drug produces a pharmacological action.

Q 11. What is absorption? Explain various mechanisms of absorption of drugs.

Absorption of Drugs

The passage of drug from route of administration into blood circulation is known as absorption.

Types/Process/Mechanism/Ways of Absorption

Absorption of drug may be either directly or indirectly but absorption involves the passage of drug dose across the cell membrane. This passage is governed by lipid carriers present at the permeable membrane. The membrane contains small pores and only water-soluble molecules can pass through them.

The absorption of drug through membrane occurs by following ways:

a. Simple Diffusion (Passive Diffusion)

- This is a bidirectional process where the rate of transfer across the membrane is proportional to the concentration ingredient of the cell membrane.
- A water-soluble drug of low molecular weight such as alcohol, urea, water itself diffuses passively through aqueous pores of the membrane.
- The drugs which are lipid soluble are mainly transferred by simple or passive diffusion after dissolution.

b. Active Transport Process

- This is a specialised process requiring energy and is independent on physical property of the membrane.
- In this process, the carrier molecule combines with drug molecule and forms a drug carrier complex on one side of the membrane.
- This complex then diffuses through the membrane and dissociates into carrier and drug molecule when reaches other side of the membrane.
- After that carrier molecule returns to the original surface to repeat the process.
- The ions which are transported by active transport process include Na^+, K^+, I^-, amino acids, some drugs, strong acids, strong bases and weak electrolytes in ionised form, glucose, pyrimidines and some antimetabolites are also transported by this process.
- This transport process is rapid than simple diffusion.

c. Pinocytosis

In this process, the cell takes up the fluid or micromolecule from its surrounding. This process is important for unicellular organisms like amoeba.

In this process, cell forms a cavity like pseudopodium and particles are taken inside the cell.

d. Filtration

The passage of drug molecule through the channels is called filtration. Small, soluble and polar drugs are absorbed by this phenomenon.

e. Facilitated Diffusion

Like passive transfer this process is also not energy-dependant. The movement of drug is from high concentration to low concentration. There is no involvement of carrier system in this process. The process is rapid than passive transport process.

Q 12. Define bioavailability. Give types of bioavailability. Give the importance or object of studying bioavailability.

Bioavailability

"It is defined as the rate and extent at which active concentration of drug is available at the desired site of action".

Types of Bioavailability

1. **Relative bioavailability:** The relative bioavailability is the bioavailability in comparison with reference standard.
2. **Absolute bioavailability:** The absolute bioavailability is the bioavailability in which whole quantity of administered drug reaches the blood circulation. It is possible only by IV route.

Study of Bioavailability is Necessary

1. To avoid toxic and side effects of the drugs.
2. To adjust the dosage regimen.
3. To study pharmacological action of drug.
4. For pre-formulation study.
5. To judge about the clinical responses of drugs.
6. To avoid wastage of drugs.
7. To decide the dose and dosage forms.

Q 13. Enumerate different factors that affect/influence the bioavailability of a drug.

Factors affecting bioavailability of drug		
a. *Pharmaceutical factors*	b. *Physiological factors*	c. *Physicochemical factors*
Dosage form	Anatomy of GIT	Particle size
Dissolution rate	Gastric emptying rate	Stability
	Gastric pH	Complex formation
	Food	Viscosity
Manufacturing variables	Interaction with GI components	Surfactants P^{KA} and P^{KB}
	First pass effect	Partition coefficient
	Diseased condition	Salt form
	Drug–drug interaction	Particle state
		Molecular weight
	GIT flora	Route of administration of drug

Q 14. Discuss physiological factors affecting (influencing) the absorption of drug (bioavailability) from the GIT or gut.

1. **Physical state of drug:** The liquids are better absorbed than solid medicaments. Aqueous solutions are more rapidly absorbed than colloids.

2. **Particle size:** Smaller the particle size, greater is the absorption of drugs from gut. Smaller particle size provides greater surface area for absorption. Thus, the dose required to produce an action is reduced due to smaller particle size.
3. **Concentration of drug:** Higher the cencentration of drug, better is the absorption of drug from intestine.
4. **Area of absorbing surface:** Larger the absorbing surface area, greater is the absorption. Thus, in small intestine the absorption of drug is greater than the stomach.
5. **Physical and mental state of the patient:** Disturbed physiological conditions such as infection, fever affect the absorption of drug. Emotional upset condition also affects absorption of drug adversely.
6. **Functional integrity of GIT:** Increased peristalsis of GIT decreases absorption of drug, e.g. in diarrhoea condition, absorption of drug decreases.
7. **pH of drug:** Acidic drugs are rapidly absorbed in stomach while basic drugs are rapidly absorbed in intestine due to respective pH ranges.
8. **Formulation:** Calcium and magnesium ions reduce the absorption of tetracyclines because tetracycline forms complexes with Ca^{++} and Mg^{++}. Hence, such formulation should not be made.
9. **Presence of other agent:** Vitamin C increases the absorption of drug from GIT. The absorption of fat-soluble vitamins increases in presence of liquid paraffin.
10. **Presence of food in GIT:** The presence of food in GIT may reduce absorption of drug from GIT because there is no direct contact with walls of GIT. But gastric irritation will not occur.
11. **First pass effect:** It is the time required for the drug to pass through hepatic portal system. The drugs are inactivated, therefore bioavailability of such drugs is reduced.

Q 15. What do you mean by distribution of drugs? Enlist various compartments in which drug is distributed. OR Write a note on 'distribution of drug in the body'.

Distribution of Drug in the Body

Distribution of drug involves transport of drug to the tissues. The body fluids act as solvents and carriers for the majority of drugs for distribution in the body. Drugs may be distributed into body as follows:

i. Extracellular fluid
ii. In blood
iii. Adipose tissue (fat)
iv. Other body tissues (organs)
v. Transcellular fluid compartments, e.g. fluids in GIT, bronchi, CSF.

- In blood, the majority of drugs are simply dissolved in serum water but some of them are bound to blood proteins such as albumin, globulin, etc.
- The plasma protein binding of drugs acts as a storage site in the blood. Thus, plasma protein binding of drug can increase the duration of action of drugs.
- Distribution of drugs into the brain and CSF depends upon the lipid soluble properties of drugs. Lipid soluble drugs enter in the brain more easily. Similarly, lipid soluble compounds cross the placental barrier and show similar pharmacological effects in both mother and foetus.
- The enterohepatic circulation is another site of drug distribution. Some drugs are extracted from the body by liver and then excreted into the small intestine via bile. Further they are reabsorbed across the mucosa back into the blood.
- Factors affecting distribution of drug in the body are:

Factors affecting drug distribution

Physiological factors
1. Cardiac output
2. Regional blood flow
3. Capillary permeability
4. Tissue volume
5. Special tissue characteristics such as blood–brain barrier

Physiochemical properties of drug
1. Binding to plasma proteins
2. Binding to other tissues like fat, liver, bone, etc.
3. Affinity for tissue constituents
4. Tissue redistribution
5. pH

The Distribution of Drugs in Specific Compartments

These are some specific compartments in the body that are characterized by barriers and they restrict entry of some drugs.

a. Blood–brain and blood–CSF barrier
b. Placental barrier.

a. BloodñBrain Barrier (BBB)

Nature has offered special protection to brain from drugs. The passage of drug in the brain is different from all organs. This is facilitated by different structure of capillaries in the CNS. Therefore only lipid soluble drugs can cross this barrier and enter inside.

Clinical significance of blood–brain barrier:

- The blood–brain barrier protects the brain from the toxic effects of lipid non-soluble drugs and poisons.
- During inflammation of meninges, permeability of BBB for drugs like penicillins or aminoglycosides is increased and they are effective.

b. Placental Barrier

Similar to BBB if also allows lipid soluble drugs but it is a weak barrier and almost all drugs can ultimately cross this barrier increases as pregnancy advances.

Distribution of Drugs in Different Body Compartments

Body compartment	*Types of drugs distributed*
1. Total body water	Small water-soluble molecules such as alcohol and antipyrine
2. Extracellular space	Large water-soluble molecules such as mannitol
3. Intracellular space	Very large, strongly protein-bound molecules such as heparin
4. Body fat	Highly lipid soluble molecules such as DDT and thiopentone
5. Bones	Fluoride and lead

Q 16. What is protein binding of drugs? Give its importance and its effects. OR Write a note on 'protein binding' of drugs.

Protein Binding of Drugs

After absorption, the drug circulates in the blood and binds with plasma proteins which is known as protein binding of drugs.

Explanation

- Due to protein binding of drug, it is not available for diffusion into extracellular compartment. Thus, there is no excretion of drug and prolongs the during of action of a drug.
- After absorption, the drug circulates in the blood either in free form or bound to plasma proteins either albumin or alpha-acid-glycoprotein.
- The fraction bound to protein usually falls as the total concentration of the drug increases and binding sites becomes saturated.
- Binding of drugs to plasma proteins assists absorption.
- Protein binding acts as a temporary 'store' of drug and tends to prevent large fluctuations in concentration of unbound drug in the body fluids.
- Protein binding reduces diffusion of the drug into the cell and thereby delays its metabolic degradation.
- Protein binding also reduces the amount of drug available for filtration at the glomeruli and hence delays its excretion.
- Protein binding reduces drug clearance.
- The extent of drug binding depends on the binding protein concentration in the plasma.

Importance of Protein Binding

1. Protein binding makes the drug inactive.
2. The drug becomes impermeable to membrane after protein.
3. Protein binding acts as a temporary storage of drugs.
4. Protein binding also reduces the amount of drug available for filtration at the glomeruli and hence reduces its excretion.
5. Protein binding reduces drug clearance.

Effects of Protein Binding on Drugs

1. Assists enteral absorption of a drug.
2. Acts as a temporary store for it and thereby prolongs drug action.
3. Causes prolonged, low levels of free drug.
4. Delays its metabolic degradation.
5. Delays its excretion.
6. Diminishes its penetration into the CNS.

Q 17. Write a note on 'biotransformation/metabolism of drugs'.

Biotransformation/Metabolism of Drugs

The alteration of drug within a living organism so as to modify its activity or its nature, is known as biotransformation or metabolism.

- The enzymes involved in the biotransformation of drugs are called microsomal enzymes.
- Some drugs are biotransformed into more active compounds, e.g.
  - i. Levodopa (inactive) is converted to dopamine (active) in brain.
  - ii. Conversion of diazepam to oxazepam which is more active.
  - iii. Conversion of phenylbutazone to oxyphenbutazone which is more active.
- The important pathways of biotransformation of drugs are:
  - i. **Oxidation:** Microsomal oxidation may involve the introduction of a hydroxyl group into the drug molecule, e.g. conversion of salicylic acid into gentisic acid.
  - ii. **Reduction:** Many halogenated compounds and nitrated aromatic compounds are reduced by the microsomal enzymes, e.g. halothane, chloramphenicol.
  - iii. **Hydrolysis:** Hydrolysis is usually carried out by enzymes esterases that hydrolyse the esters.

    Drugs like pethidine, procaine, acetylcholine are hydrolysed by esterase.
  - iv. **Conjugation:** This is a synthetic process by which a drug or its metabolite is combined with an endogenous substance, resulting in various conjugates such as glucuronides, etheral sulphates and amino acid conjugates, e.g. phenobarbitone is oxidised to its hydroxy derivative which is conjugated with glucuronic acid.

Factors Affecting Drug Metabolism/Biotransformation

1. Animal species and strains
2. Age and sex
3. Genetic determinants
4. Nutritional status
5. Altitude and temperature
6. Route and duration of drug administration
7. Environmental determinants such as air solution

8. Simultaneous administration of other drugs
9. Presence of disease (hepatic/renal damage)

Q 18. Define metabolism/biotransformation. Mention the enzymes responsible for metabolism of drugs. Explain types of biotransformation reactions.

Metabolism /Biotransformation

The alteration of drug within a living organism so as to modify its activity or nature, is known as biotransformation or metabolism.

Enzymes for Biotransformation

a. **Microsomal enzymes:** They are present in the smooth endoplasmic reticulum of the liver, kidney and GIT, e.g. glucuronyl transferase, dehydrogenase, hydroxylase and cytochrome P450.

b. **Non-microsomal enzymes:** They are present in the cytoplasm, mitochondria of different organs, e.g. esterases, amidase, hydrolase.

Types of Biotransformation Reactions

1. Phase 1 Reactions (Non-synthetic Reactions)

- In this phase, the enzymes carryout oxidation, reduction and hydrolysis reactions.
- The phase 1 reactions introduce functional groups such as –OH, –COOH, –SH, –O–, $-NH_2$, etc.
- The phase 1 reactions leads to inactivation of active drug.
- The phase 1 reaction is reffered as functionalisation phase of drug metabolism.
- Phase 1 reactions are carried out by CYPs (cytochrome P450 isoenzyme), flavin-containing monooxygenases (FMO) and epoxide hydrolases (EH).

a. **Oxidation:** Microsomal oxidation involves the introduction of an oxygen or removal of hydrogen atom.

b. **Reduction:** The reduction reaction will take place by the enzyme reductase which catalyze the reduction of azo and nitro compounds, e.g. prontosil converted to sulfonamide.

c. **Hydrolysis:** Hydrolysis is usually carried out by the enzymes esterases that hydrolyse the esters, e.g. drugs like pethidine, procaine, acetylcholine are hydrolysed by esterase.

2. Phase 2 Reactions (Synthetic Reactions/Conjugation Reactions)

This is a synthetic process by which a drug or its metabolite is combined with an endogenous substance, resulting in various conjugates such as glucuronides, etheral sulphates and amino acid conjugates.

The active enzymes in this phase 2 reaction include UDP-glucuronosyl-transferases (UGT), sulfotransferases, glutathione-S transferases (GST), e.g. phenobarbitone is oxidised to its hydroxy derivative which is conjugated with glucuronic acid.

Q 19. What is 'disposition/excretion' of drugs? Explain different routes/channels/ways of excretion of drugs from the body. OR Write a note on 'disposition/excretion of drugs'.

Excretion/Disposition of Drugs (Elimination of Drugs)

It means removal of a drug from the body through various routes.

The important channels of excretion of drugs are as follows:

1. **Kidney:** The kidneys act as a primary organ for the excretion of most of the drugs. The rate of glomerular filtrate, tubular reabsorption and tubular secretion influences the rate of excretion of drugs, e.g. weak acids are quickly eliminated in an alkaline urine while weak bases are rapidly excreted in an acidic urine.
2. **Lungs:** Volatile general anaesthetics and certain other drugs like paraldehyde and alcohol are partially excreted by the lungs.
3. **Skin:** Some metals like arsenic and mercury may be partly excreted through the skin. Arsenic gets deposited in the hair follicles on prolonged administration. This phenomenon is useful for detecting arsenic poisoning.
4. **Bile:** The drugs such as erythromycin are excreted in the urine only in small amounts but appear in high concentration in bile and are partially excreted into the intestine through the bile.
5. **Intestine:** Some substances which are not fully absorbed from the GIT are excreted in the faeces, e.g. purgatives like senna.
6. **Milk:** Antibiotics are deposited in the milk. Drugs like chloramphenicol, chlorpromazine, diazepam are deposited in milk and excreted via milk.
7. **Saliva:** Certain drugs like iodides and metallic salts are excreted in the saliva. Lead compounds deposited as lead sulphide produce blue line on gums.

Q 20. Define pharmacodynamics. Explain various general mechanisms of action of a drug.

Pharmacodynamics

It is the study of mechanism of action of drug and the pharmacological effects produced on the human body.

General Mechanisms of Action of a Drug/Types of Drug Actions

The drug may produce their effects by following different mechanisms:

1. By stimulation
2. By depression
3. By irritation
4. By replacement of a deficient hormone.
5. As anti-infective agents
6. By modification of the immune status.

1. By Stimulation

- Increase in activity of specialized cells is called stimulation.
- Excess stimulation produces changes in the protoplasm of the cell which may ultimately leads to depression.
- A drug may specifically stimulate certain portion of a particular system but depress others, e.g. morphine stimulates the vagus and the oculomotor nuclei and chemoreceptor trigger zone but depresses the respiratory and cough centres.

2. By Depression

- Decrease in the activity of specialized cells is called depression.
- Quinine depresses the myocardium while barbiturate depresses the central nervous system.

3. By Irritation

- The term irritation indicates that a drug produces adverse effects on the growth, nutrition and morphology of living tissues.
- Irritation is thus a phenomenon not restricted to specialized cells but can occur in all the body tissues.
- Irritation produces changes in the cellular structure and is capable of producing inflammation, corrosion and necrosis of cells.

a. Astringent effect (precipitation of proteins)
b. Dehydration
c. Action on cellular enzymes, usually inhibition
d. Cytotoxic action
e. Counter irritant action (e.g. like turpentine oil)

4. By Replacement of a Deficient Hormone

- In this case drugs may be used as replacement when the production of endogenous substance is reduced.
- Replacement finds an important application in the treatment of hormonal deficiencies, e.g. insulin in diabetes mellitus.

5. As Anti-infective Agents

The drugs are used for prevention, arrest and eradication of infections, they act specifically on the causative organisms.

6. Modification of Immune Status

Vaccine, sera and certain other agents act by altering the immune status.

Q 21. Enlist various factors modifying drug action.

1. Body weight
2. Age
3. Sex
4. Route of administration
5. Time of administration
6. Diet and environmental factor
7. Genetic factor
8. Emotional factor
9. Presence of disease
10. Metabolic disturbances
11. Cumulative effect
12. Additive effect
13. Synergism (potentiation)
14. Antagonism
15. Tolerance
16. Dependance.

Q 22. Explain the factors modifying drug action.

1. **Body weight:** The dose of a drug is related to body weight. The dose of drug is usually expressed as mg/kg of body weight.
2. **Age:** Infants and old patients need dose different from adults. In infants, the metabolising enzymes and excretory process are not fully developed. Hence, doses of children should be smaller than adults.
3. **Sex:** Some drugs which cross the placental barrier and depress foetal respiration are avoided in pregnant women, e.g. morphine.
4. **Route of administration of drug:** As the route of administration changes, the dose required for same pharmacological action varies. Hence, IV dose is smaller than SC dose which is smaller than oral dose.

   IV dose < SC dose < oral dose.
5. **Time of administration of drugs:** When the drugs are taken before meals, the absorption is greater, but there is irritation to GIT due to direct contact of drug with walls of GIT.

   When the drugs are taken after meals, the absorption is poor but there is not irritation to GIT. This is because drug is mixed with food material hence direct contact of drug with walls of GIT is avoided.
6. **Diet and environmental factor:** In the presence of diet, the absorption of drug is poor. Environmental factor also affects the variations in the doses of drugs, e.g.
   i. The alcohol is well tolerated in cold environment than in summer.
   ii. The dose of phenobarbitone required to produce a sleep during day-time is much more than the dose required during night.
7. **Genetic factor:** The patients with hereditary metabolic disorders rarely show a disturbance in the metabolism of drugs. This is because of microsomal enzyme systems involved in the metabolism of drugs. Thus, the genetic factor gives individual variations in response to drugs. Some drugs pass through genes and modify drug response from generation to generation, e.g. diabetes mellitus.

8. **Emotional factor:** The personality of the physician may influence the drug effect particularly in psychic patients. Hence, nervous patients require smaller doses of drugs as compared to normal patients.
9. **Presence of disease:** In diseased conditions, some drugs may produce unusually prolonged effects in cirrhotic patients. Thus, drugs like barbiturates and chlorpromazine may produce unusually prolonged effects in cirrhotic patients.
10. **Metabolic disturbances:** The changes in water balance, electrolyte balance and acid–base balance, body temperature and other physiological factors may modify the effects of drugs, e.g. the absorption of iron from the GIT is maximum if the individual has an iron deficiency anaemia.
11. **Cumulation (cumulative effect):** When excretion of drug is slow, repeated administration of drug accumulates in the body and may lead to toxicity. This is known as cumulation. The phenomenon is known as cumulative effect, e.g. digitalis, emetine, heavy metals, chloramphenicol show cumulation.
    Cumulation can be avoided by following ways:
    i. Stop the administration of drug at the appearance of first warning symptom.
    ii. It must be known that the drug is eliminated slowly or rapidly.
    iii. Carefully select the dosage form in which the drug is to be administered.
    iv. Check the liver and kidney function before and during drug administration.
12. **Additive effect:** When total pharmacological action of two or more drugs administered together is equivalent to their individual pharmacological actions, the phenomenon is known as additive effect, i.e.
    $$1 + 1 = 2$$
    For example, combination of ephedrine and aminophylline shows additive effect in the treatment of bronchial asthma.
13. **Synergistic effect (synergism):** The increase in pharmacological response by the use of two or more drugs at the same time is called synergism. The effect is known as synergistic effect, i.e.
    $$1 + 1 = 3$$
    For example:
    a. Aspirin and codeine as analgesic
    b. Sulphamethoxazole and trimethoprim as antibacterial
    c. Aspirin, phenacetin and caffeine as analgesic.
14. **Antagonism:** The opposite actions of two drugs on the same physiological system are termed antagonism.

- *Classification/types of antagonism*
  i. **Chemical antagonism:** When the biological activity of drug is totally reduced by a chemical reaction with another agent, the phenomenon is known as chemical antagonism, e.g. acid and alkali react with each other for neutralization.

ii. **Competitive/reversible antagonism:** In competitive antagonism, the agonist and antagonist compete for the same receptor. Hence, in such cases, the extent to which the antagonist opposes the pharmacological action of agonist depends on the relative number of receptors occupied by two compounds, e.g. acetylcholine and atropine compete for each other at the receptor sites.

If concentration of acetylcholine is increased, the blockade produced by atropine can be overcome. Hence, antagonism is also termed reversible antagonism.

iii. **Noncompetitive irreversible antagonism:** In this type of antagonism, the antagonist inactivates the receptor by some mechanism in such a way that the effective complex with agonist cannot be formed. Hence, though the concentration of agonist is increased at the receptor site, the receptor is inactive to produce any combination with agonist. Hence, there is no any pharmacological action with agonist. Thus, it is called irreversible antagonism, e.g. acetylcholine and papaverine on smooth muscles produce noncompetitive antagonism.

iv. **Physiological antagonism:** When a drug is administered, it reverses the effects of another drug by acting on different receptors. This phenomenon is known as physiological antagonism, e.g. adrenaline and histamine reactions are of this type.

v. **Functional antagonism:** When interaction of two agonists which act independently of each other but give opposite effects take place, the reaction is known as functional antagonism, e.g. acetylcholine and adrenaline show functional antagonism.

• **Importance of antagonism**

i. Antagonism is useful in poisoning cases to block the actions of poisons.
ii. Antagonism is useful to control the adverse effects of the drugs.
iii. Antagonism is useful to adjust the doses of the drugs combined.

15. **Drug tolerance:** When large dose of a drug is required to get an effect, produced by the normal therapeutic dose of a drug, the phenomenon is known as drug tolerance.

• **Types/classification of tolerance**

A. **True tolerance:** It is seen on both oral and parenteral administration.

a. ***Natural tolerance:*** It results in difference between species and races.

i. *Species tolerance:* Some animal species can tolerate large amount of particular drug which may prove to be lethal (toxic) to man, e.g. some rabbits can tolerate large amount of belladonna. This is because of enzyme atropine esterase present in the rabbits' liver and plasma which rapidly detoxify the belladonna.

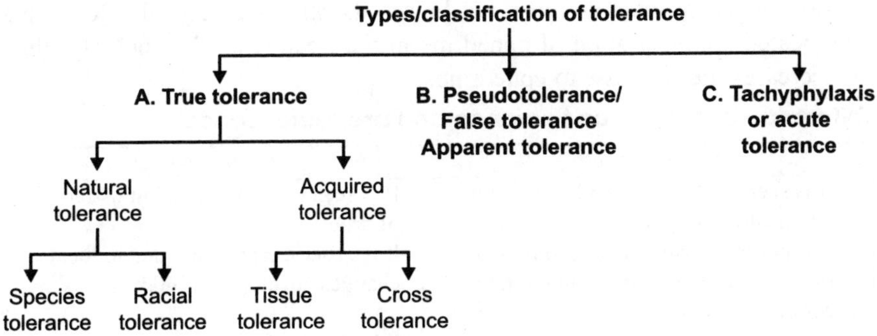

ii. *Racial tolerance:* When solution of ephedrine is instilled into the conjunctival sac of the Caucasians, it produces prompt dilation of pupils but in Negroes ephedrine does not produce any dilation at all.

b. ***Acquired tolerance:*** Repeated administration of drug produce a tendency to produce a tolerance. This is known as acquired tolerance, e.g. the drugs like barbiturates, opiates, alcohol, xanthines, produce acquired type of tolerance. Acquired tolerance is of two types:

i. *Tissue tolerance:* In this type, development of tolerance is related to certain pharmacological action and certain tissues, organs or systems, e.g. morphine produces tolerance for its euphoriant effect but pupils and GIT never become tolerated. Thus, same dose of morphine invariably produces constipation but may fail to "euphoria".

ii. *Cross tolerance:* When an individual develops tolerance to a drug belonging to a particular group, it also shows tolerance to other drugs belonging to the same grouping, it is known as cross tolerance, e.g. tolerance to vasodialator effect of 'glyceryl trinitrite' in an individual shows tolerance to 'pentaerythritol tetranitrite' which belongs to same group.

B. **Pseudotolerance/false/apparent tolerance:** It is observed only by oral route. When small dose of poison is taken orally, tolerance is developed to that poison by the GIT. This is possible after repeated administration of small quantity by oral route in the individual immune to such poison.

This tolerance to the oral administration of drug is probably due to local changes developed by GIT which prevent poison from getting absorbed into the systemic circulation.

C. **Tachyphylaxis/acute tolerance:** The repeated administration of drug within a short interval of time decreases the pharmacological response progressively. This phenomenon is known as tachyphylaxis or acute tolerance.

Tachyphylaxis probably can occur if the drug dissociates only slowly from its combination with receptor and thus continuing receptor blockade, while loosing its intrinsic activity, i.e. looses its pharmacological effects, e.g. repeated administration of ephedrine in the treatment of bronchial asthma decreases the response to ephedrine.

Difference between true tolerance and pseudotolerance

True tolerance	*Pseudotolerance*
1. It is seen on both oral and parenteral administration of drug	It is seen only on oral administration of drug
2. It is observed naturally due to presence of certain enzyme system to tolerate certain drugs	It is observed probably due to local changes developed by GIT
3. It is further divided into: i. Natural tolerance, ii. Acquired tolerance	It has no further types
4. Example, morphine produces tolerance for its euphoriant effect but pupils and GIT are not affected	Example, if small quantity of poison is taken orally, poisoning will not occur

16. **Drug dependance:** It is a psychic or physical condition of the person due to interaction between living organism and drug, which includes a compulsion to take the drug and tendency to increase the dose at the cost of health, e.g. morphine, heroin, alcohol, tobacco.

- Dependance is of two types:
   i. *Physical dependance:* It is the condition in which the body shows dependant stage on the drug. If the drug is withdrawn, the intense physical disturbances occur.
   ii. *Psychic dependance:* A condition in which a drug produces a feeling of satisfaction and a psychic drive that requires periodic or continuous administration of the drug to produce pleasure and to avoid discomfort is called psychic dependance.

Q 23. Give the formulae for calculating doses in children.

a. Age-based Formulae

1. Young's formula $\text{Child dose} = \dfrac{\text{Age in years}}{\text{Age in years}+12} \times \text{Adult dose}$
2. WJ Dilling formula $\text{Child dose} = \dfrac{\text{Age in years}}{20} \times \text{Adult dose}$
3. Fried's rule for infant $\text{Infant dose} = \dfrac{\text{Age in months}}{150} \times \text{Adult dose}$

b. Body Weight-based Formulae

1. Clark's formula $\text{Child dose} = \dfrac{\text{Wt of child in kg}}{70} \times \text{Adult dose}$
2. Clark's rule for infants $\text{Dose of infant} = \dfrac{\text{Wt in pound}}{150} \times \text{Adult dose}$

c. As per Surface Area $\frac{\text{Surface area of child (m}^2)}{\text{Surface area of adult (m}^2)\ (1.73\text{m}^2)} \times 100 = \%$ of adult dose

Q 24. Give the difference between 'drug tolerance and tachyphylaxis'.

Drug tolerance	*Tachyphylaxis*
1. It develops slowly	It develops rapidly
2. It takes a time-in days to months	It develops within a few minutes
3. The higher dose causes tolerance	It does not depend on dose
4. The effects are seen when dose is increased	The effects are not seen even when dose is increased
5. Seen routinely in clinical practice	Not seen routinely in clinical practice
6. For example: Opium, barbiturates, ethanol, etc.	Frequent administration of ephedrine in bronchial asthma

Q 25. Define 'therapeutic index' (TI). Give the reasons 'why a drug with larger therapeutic index is safer than one with smaller therapeutic index'. OR 'Drugs having lesser therapeutic index should be administered cautiously'. OR 'Why therapeutic index shows margin of safety of drug'?

Therapeutic Index

Therapeutic index is the ratio of median lethal dose (LD_{50}) and median effective dose (ED_{50}).

$$\text{Therapeutic index (TI)} = \frac{LD_{50}}{ED_{50}}$$

Reason

1. Therapeutic index indicates the relative margin of safety of a drug.
2. A dose of the drug which produces the stated effect in 50% of individuals within the population is called median dose.
3. Depending upon the stated effect it can be designated as 'median effective dose (ED_{50}) and median lethal dose (LD_{50})'.
4. The therapeutic index indicates how close the effective dose is to the lethal dose for 50% of the test population. Thus, therapeutic index gives an idea about the 'margin of safety'.
5. As the ED_{50} approaches the ED_{50}, the danger of the drug toxicity increases significantly.
6. Therefore, a drug with larger therapeutic index is safer than one with smaller therapeutic index. Hence, drug with lesser therapeutic index should be administered cautiously.
7. Therefore therapeutic index shows margin of safety of drug.
8. Drugs with a therapeutic index of 10 or more are almost sure to be safe.

Objective Questions with Answers in Bold Letters

1. **Pharmacology** is the science, which deals with the drugs and their actions on human body or animals.
2. **Pharmacodynamics** is concerned with study of mechanism of action of drugs and pharmacological effects produced on the human body.
3. **Pharmacokinetic** includes the study of absorption, distribution, metabolism and excretion of drugs.
4. **Toxicology** is the science deals with study of poisons.
5. **Posology** deals with the study of doses of drugs.
6. **Teratology** is a branch of science which concern with the harmful effects of drugs on foetus.
7. Pharmacokinetics decides the **fate of drug** in the body.
8. In **sublingual** route tablets are placed under the tongue.
9. Maximum **10 ml** volume of drug can be administered by intramuscular (IM) route.
10. Accurate blood levels of drug can be achieved only by **intravenous route**.
11. The routes of administration of drugs other than alimentary canal are called **parenteral routes.**
12. 100% bioavailability is possible only by **intravenous route**.
13. **Intradermal route** is useful for the detection of drug allergy.
14. Injections with oily bases can be given by **intramuscular route**.
15. In **iontophoresis**, the galvanic current is used for penetration of drug into the deeper tissues.
16. Certain drugs are rubbed into the skin to get absorbed and produce systemic effect, the route is known as **innuction.**
17. Enema preparations, suppositories are administered by **rectal route**.
18. A drug which combines with receptor and produces a pharmacological response is called **agonist**.
19. A drug which combines with receptor is called **antagonist**.
20. The ability of a drug to combine with receptor is known as **affinity** of a drug for the receptor.
21. The ability of a drug to give a pharmacological action after combination with the receptor is called **efficacy (instrinsic activity)**.
22. The **absorption** means passage of drug from route or administration into the blood circulation.
23. Simple diffusion (passive diffusion) is a **bidirectional** process.
24. The energy is required for **active transport process** of absorption of drug.
25. In **pinocytosis**, the drug molecules/particles are taken inside the cell in cavity like pseudopodium.
26. In **first pass effect**, the drugs go to liver first and then into the blood circulation.

27. **Bioavailability** means the rate and extent at which the active concentration of drug reaches in blood and is available at the desired site of action.
28. **Distribution** of drug involves the transport of drug to the tissues.
29. Distribution of drugs in the brain and CSF depends upon the **lipid soluble** properties of drug.
30. BBB means **blood–brain barrier**.
31. **Protein binding** acts as a temporary storage of drug.
32. Protein binding makes the drug **inactive**.
33. Protein binding produced **prolonged** drug actions.
34. **Biotransformation/metabolism** involves modification of activity or nature of drug.
35. The enzymes involved in the biotransformation of drugs are called **microsomal enzymes**.
36. **Disposition/elimination** means removal of drug from the body through various routes.
37. The accumulation/deposition of drug in the body producing toxicity is known as **cumulation**.
38. When total pharmacological action of two or more drugs administered together is equivalent to their individual pharmacological actions, the phenomenon is known as **additive effect**.
39. **Synergism/synergistic** effect means increase in pharmacological effect by the use of two or more drugs at the same time.
40. The opposite actions of two drugs on the same physiological system, the phenomenon is known as **antagonism**.
41. **Theapeutic index** indicates the relative 'margin of safety' of a drug.
42. The drugs with **larger** therapeutic index are safer.
43. The drugs having **lesser** therapeutic index should be administered cautiously.
44. Only up to **2 ml** quantity of drug can be injected by subcutaneous route.
45. Total volume of drug injected by intramuscular route is restricted up to **10 ml**.
46. In **intramedullary injection route** the drugs are directly injected into the bone marrow.
47. **Enteral route** means the drug is placed directly in the gastrointestinal tract (GIT).
48. The effect produced by the drug after being effectively where it is absorbed in blood stream is known as **systemic effect**.
49. The effect produced by the drug in a localized area where it is applied is known as **local effect**.
50. A **receptor** is a specific functional cellular component which when combines with drug produces a pharmacological action.
51. **Phase 1 reaction** of biotransformation is known as non-synthetic reaction.
52. **Cytochrome P450** is a microsomal enzyme involved in biotransformation reactions.

53. The phase 1 reaction of biotransformation leads to **inactivation** of active drug.
54. The phase 1 reaction is reffered as **functionalisation** phase of drug metabolism/biotransformation.
55. The phase 2 reaction is also known as **synthetic reaction/conjugation reaction**.
56. **UDP–glucuronosyltransferases (UGT)** is active enzyme involved in phase 2 reaction of biotransformation.
57. **Pharmacokinetics** is the movement or passage of drug across the body.
58. The process which refers to the passage of a drug dose over cell membrane from the point of delivery to the bloodstream is called **absorption**.
59. The primary site of drug metabolism is **liver**.
60. Simple diffusion is also called **passive diffusion**.
61. The macromolecules with which medicines bind to elicit their specific biological effects are called **receptors**.
62. The phenomenon of two medications being used at the same time to facilitate pharmacological action is called **synergism**.

Chapter 2

Drugs Acting on Peripheral Nervous System

- Cholinergic drugs/parasympathomimetics
- Adrenergics
- Neuromuscular blocking agents
- Local anaesthetic agents
- Anticholinergic
- Antiadrenergics
- Drugs used in myasthenia gravis
- Nonsteroidal anti-inflammatory drugs (NSAIDs)

INTRODUCTION

I. Divisions of Nervous System

The nervous system

- Central nervous system (CNS)
- Peripheral nervous system (PNS)
  - Somatic nervous system (controls voluntary motor functions)
  - Autonomic nervous system (controls involuntary automatic functions)
    - Sympathetic nervous system (SNS)
    - Parasympathetic nervous system (PSNS)

II. Fundamental Steps involved in Neurohumoral Transmission

Synthesis of transmitters

↓

Storage of transmitters

↓

Release and transmitters by nerve action potential

↓

Interaction of the released transmitters with receptors and the effector cell

↓

Rapid removal of the transmitter

↓

Recovery and the effector cell into previous state

III. Divisions of ANS (Autonomic Nervous System)

Drugs acting on ANS

- Sympathetic nervous system
  - Sympathomimetics (adrenergics) e.g. adrenaline, isoprenaline, ephedrine, amphetamine
  - Sympatholytics (antiadrenergics) e.g. tolazoline, labetalol, propranolol, atenolol
- Parasympathetic nervous system
  - Parasympathomimetics (cholinergics) e.g. acetylcholine, carbachol, physostigmine, neostigmine
  - Parasympatholytics (anticholinergics) e.g. atropine, hyoscine, benzatropine, homatropine

A. CHOLINERGIC DRUGS/PARASYMPATHOMIMETICS

Q 1. Define and classify cholinergic drugs with examples.

Cholinergic Drugs

The drugs that stimulate the parasympathetic nervous system are called cholinergics/parasympathomimetics/cholinomimetics/cholinergic agonists.

- These drugs mimic the effect of acetylcholine.
- Acetylcholine is neurotransmitter for parasympathetic nervous system.

Classification of Cholinergic Drugs/Parasympathomimetics

1. Direct Acting

a. Cholinomimetic alkaloids, e.g. pilocarpine, muscarine, arecholine, nicotine.
b. Esters of choline, e.g. acetylcholine, carbachol, methacholine, bethanechol.

2. Indirect Acting (Anticholinesterase/cholinesterase Inhibitors)

a. Reversible, e.g. physostigmine, neostigmine, pyridostigmine, edrophonium.
b. Irreversible, e.g. organophosphates, parathione, dyflos.

Q 2. Describe pharmacological actions of acetylcholine/cholinergic drugs.

Acetylcholine

It is an ester of choline with acetic acid. Its actions are divided into:

a. *Muscarinic actions:* By stimulation of muscarinic receptors which are similar to mushroom alkaloid muscarine.
b. *Nicotinic actions:* By stimulation of nicotinic receptors which are similar to nicotine alkaloid from tobacco.

a. Muscarinic Actions of Acetylcholine

1. **On heart:** Acetylcholine depresses the activity of SA node and reduces the heart rate and may produce cardiac arrest.

Acetylcholine decreases the cardiac contractility and automaticity, rhythmicity and conductivity.

2. **On blood vessels:** Acetylcholine dilates the blood vessels and causes decrease in peripheral resistance and output and leads to hypotension.
3. **Smooth muscles of GIT:** Acetylcholine increases the rhythmic activity of smooth muscles of GIT and increases peristalsis. Acetylcholine contracts smooth muscles of gallbladder and urinary bladder.
4. **Secretions:** Acetylcholine increases the gastric, intestinal, bronchial, salivary, lacrimal secretions. Acetylcholine increases sweating.
5. **On eye:** Acetylcholine produces constriction of pupil (miosis).

b. Nicotinic Actions of Acetylcholine

Acetylcholine produces nicotinic actions on autonomic ganglia, adrenal medulla, motor end plates of skeletal muscles.

1. Acetylcholine stimulates the adrenal medulla to release adrenaline and noradrenaline.
2. Acetylcholine induces contraction of skeletal muscles.

Q 3. Write in brief about 'methacholine' and carbachol.

1. Methacholine

It differs from acetylcholine in the following respects:

a. It can be administered orally.
b. It is comparatively resistant to true cholinesterase and totally resistant to pseudocholinesterase.
c. The duration of action is longer.
d. It has selective cholinergic actions, which include mainly muscarinic actions and no or very weak nicotinic actions.
e. Amongst muscarinic actions the effects on smooth muscles of GIT are prominent.

The drug produces transient hypotension, tachycardia, salivation, sweating and flushing. It increases intestinal and pancreatic secretions. It may produce bronchospasm.

Therapeutic uses/Indications: It was formerly used to treat myasthenia gravis and to test for the presence or absence of pheochrome tumors. It is rarely used clinically these days. Earlier when used, it was given subcutaneously in the dose of 10 to 25 mg.

2. Carbachol

Carbachol is more potent than methacholine and is resistant to both true and pseudochlinesterase. It is better absorbed in gastrointestinal tract as compared to other esters of choline.

Pharmacological Actions: It has selective muscarinic effect on smooth muscles of gastrointestinal tract. It also stimulates autonomic ganglia and skeletal muscles.

In therapeutic doses, it produces flushing of the face, sweating, salivation and lacrimation. It may produce increased desire for micturition and defaecation. The muscarinic effects of carbachol are not effectively antagonished by atropine.

Therapeutic uses/Indications

- It was fomerly used in gastroenterology and genitourinary practice.
- Today it is used in ophthalmology for the treatment of glaucoma in the form of eye drops.

Q 4. Describe the pharmacological actions and uses of neostigmine.

Neostigmine

It is a reversible anticholinesterase.

- It inhibits both true and pseudocholinesterases.

Pharmacological Actions

Some important pharmacological actions of neostigmine are as follows:

1. **Gastrointestinal system:** It improves the tone and motility of the gut, as well as peristalsis and gastric juice production. It also aids in the movement of digestive contents.
2. **Skeletal muscles:** In patients with myasthenia gravis, it increases the strength of their skeletal muscles (skeletal muscle fatigue at the end of the day). This is because of its anticholinesterase properties, which cause a buildup of ACh in motor end plates. During each nerve impulse, the amount of acetylcholine released increases. Because acetylcholine's partial agonist action, it can directly stimulate cholinergic receptors.
3. **Cardiovascular system:** By causing peripheral vasodilation, the medication lowers blood pressure and lowers heart rate. The stimulation of sympathetic ganglia counteracts this effect. As a result, the drug's effect on the cardiovascular system is dependent on a number of complex elements and thus unpredictable.
4. **Eye:** The medication causes miosis, accommodation spasms and a drop in intraocular tension when it is injected locally into the eye.

5. **Autonomic ganglia:** The medication stimulates the autonomic ganglia at low concentrations while blocking them at high quantities.
6. **Miscellaneous:** It stimulates different secretions and causes bronchial constriction, just like other cholinergic medications.

Therapeutic uses

1. In the treatment of glaucoma.
2. In the treatment of myasthenia gravis.
3. In the treatment of postoperative paralytic ileus.
4. In the treatment of paroxysmal atrial tachycardia.

Dosage: Neostigmine bromide oral tablet 15 mg.

Q 5. Give the signs, symptoms and treatments of organophosphorus compound poisoning.

Organophosphorus Compound Poisoning

The poisoning with organophosphorus compounds may be due to:

a. Occupational, as in persons engaged in spraying insecticides.
b. Accidental, by consumption of agricultural products sprayed with insecticide.
c. Suicidal, due to intentional ingestion.

Signs and Symptoms

1. Miosis
2. Headache
3. Bronchospasm
4. Hypotension
5. Respiratory depression
6. Convulsions
7. Nausea, vomiting
8. Abdominal cramps
9. Anorexia
10. Diarrhoea.

Treatments

1. If ingestion is by mouth, rapid gastric lavage is advised.
2. Mouth and pharyngeal secretions are removed by suction.
3. For removal of secretions and maintenance of patient's airway, place the patient in a proper position.
4. Endotracheal intubation is necessary for proper respiration.
5. If the body is soiled with insectides, remove clothes and give medicated bath.
6. Drug treatment
   a. Atropine sulphate 2 to 4 mg initially up to 50 mg parenterally to block all secretions.
   b. Enzyme reactivators such as pralidoxamine (2-PAM) 1 to 2 gm by slow IV injection.
   c. Convulsions may be controlled by injecting trimethadione 1 gm after every 15 minutes.

Q 6. Give the dose, route, brand name and uses of the following cholinergic drugs.

Cholinergic Drugs

Drug	*Brand name*	*Uses*	*Dose*	*Route*
i. Methacholine	Mecholyl	Paroxysmal tachycardia, for diagnosis of belladonna poisoning	10–40 mg	SC
ii. Carbachol	Carbachol	For postoperative paralytic ileus, for urinary retention	0.25–0.5 mg 1–4 mg	SC Oral
iii. Bethanechol	ACh	To treat abdominal distension, paralytic ileus, postoperative urinary retention	2.5–30 mg 30–100 mg	SC Oral
iv. Acetylcholine	ACh	In combination with mannitol is used for constriction of pupil	1% solution of acetylcholine chloride with 5% mannitol	Local
v. Pilocarpine	Pilocar Carpomiotic	**Uses:** 1. In an open angle glaucoma 2. As a miotic 3. To control mydriasis and cycloplegia 4. To break adhesion between iris and lens along with mydriatics	1–5% solution	Eye drop
vi. Neostigmine	Prostigmine	In myaesthenia gravis, paralytic ileus, postoperative urinary retention	60–120 mg 0.25–1 mg	Oral SC or IM
vii. Physostigmine	Eserine	1. As a miotic, in glaucoma 2. To treat atropine poisoning	60–180 mg 1–5 mg	Oral SC or IM

B. ANTICHOLINERGICS

Q 1. Define and classify anticholinergics/parasympatholytics.

Anticholinergics

The drugs which blocks the actions produced by stimulation of parasympathetic nervous system are called anticholinergics.

Anticholinergics are also known as parasympatholytics or cholinergic antagonists, cholinergic blockers.

Classification

1. Belladonna alkaloids: Atropine, hyoscine (scopolamine).
2. Semisynthetic derivative: Homatropine, ipratropine bromide.
3. Synthetic compounds: Propantheline, oxyphenonium, dicyclomine, cyclopentolate.

Q 2. Give the mechanism of action, pharmacological actions, therapeutic uses, adverse effects of atropine.

Atropine

It is an alkaloid obtained from *Atropa belladonna*.

Mechanism of Action: Atropine competitively antagonises acetylcholine at muscarinic receptor. Atropine has a greater affinity for the muscarinic receptors than does acteylcholine but lacks efficacy in initiating activity. It does not interfere with release of acetylcholine at cholinergic sites. Thus, the nicotinic actions of acetylcholine at autonomic ganglia and voluntary muscles remain unaltered. The muscarinic blockade produced by atropine can be reversed by increasing the concentration of acetylcholine at the muscarinic cholinergic sites.

Pharmacological Actions

1. **On GIT:** Atropine reduces tone, motility or peristalsis of GIT and produces constipation.
2. **On CVS:** In larger doses, atropine increases heart rate (tachycardia).
3. **Urinary tract:** Atropine reduces the movements of ureters and urinary bladder and tends to produce urinary retention.
4. **On CNS:** In larger doses, atropine produces marked CNS stimulation which may cause restlessness, irritability, disorientation.
5. **On eye:** Atropine has two primary effects on the eye, i.e. mydriasis (dilation of pupil) and cycloplegia (paralysis of accommodation).
6. **On secretions:** Atropine reduces all exocrine secretions including lacrimal, salivary, gastric, intestinal, laryngeal, pharyngeal and causes dryness of mouth and intense thirst. Hence, also called antisecretory agent.

On local instillation, atropine produces mydriasis by blocking the cholinergic nerve supply. The ciliary muscles of the eye are likewise paralysed by atropine which causes increase in focal length of the lens. Thus, individual can see the things only at long distance. This is termed "cycloplegia".

As the muscles of sphincter of iris are paralysed, individual cannot constrict the pupil in response to bright light. Because of mydriasis and cycloplegia, person fails to respond to bright light, this is known as "photophobia".

Adverse Effects

1. Dryness of mouth and intense thirst
2. Blurring of vision (photophobia)
3. Constipation
4. Difficulty in swallowing
5. Retention of urine
6. Palpitation, tachycardia
7. Hyperpyrexia
8. Dermatitis

Therapeutic uses

1. As antispasmodics
2. In peptic ulcer
3. As a preanaesthetic medication
4. To produce mydriasis and cycloplegia
5. In organophosphorus poisoning
6. In parkinsonism
7. In motion sickness
8. In myocardial infarction.

Dosage: Atropine tablet 0.6–1.2 mg for oral administration.
Brand name: Tropine

Contraindications

- Myasthenia gravis
- Paralytic ileus
- Prostate enlargement.

Q 3. Give signs, symptoms and treatments of 'acute atropine poisoning'. OR Write a note on 'acute atropine poisoning/acute belladonna poisoning'.

Acute Atropine Poisoning/Acute Belladonna Poisoning

The poisoning with atropine is caused due to overdosing of atropine during treatment or ingestion of leaves or seeds of belladonna.

Signs and Symptoms

1. Dryness of mouth
2. Mydriasis
3. Blurring of vision and photophobia
4. Urinary retention
5. Hyperpyrexia
6. Restlessness
7. Slurring of speech
8. Intense thirst
9. Difficulty in swallowing
10. Mania and delirium

Treatments

1. If the poisoning is by mouth, to remove the poison gastric lavage is advised.
2. Dark room is given to the patient to relieve photophobia.
3. Catheterisation is advised for management of urinary retention.
4. To treat hyperpyrexia ice cold sponging is advised.
5. Artificial respiration is advised.
6. To treat delirium and restlessness, diazepam is given.
7. Good nursing care is essential.
8. Alkaloidal inactivators such as universal antidotes are given before and after gastric lavage.
9. Physostigmine (1–4 mg) is given intravenously as it rapid blocks the central effects of atropine.

Q 4. Give the uses, dose, route, brand names and adverse effect of the following anticholinergics.

Anticholinergic Drugs

Drug	*Brand name*	*Dose*	*Route*	*Major adverse effect*
1. Atropine	Tropine	0.6–2 mg/ml	IM/IV	Photophobia
2. Scopolamine (hyoscine)	Hystalin, hytrol	2.5 mg	Oral, IM	Dryness of mouth, blurring of vision

C. ADRENERGICS

Q 1. Define and classify adrenergics/sympathomimetics.

Adrenergics

The drugs which nimic the responses obtained by stimulation of sympathetic nervous system are called adrenergics.

Classification

- On basis of catechol nucleus
  - i. Catecholamines, e.g. adrenaline, noradrenaline, isoprenaline.
  - ii. Noncatecholamines, e.g. ephedrine, amphetamine, salbutamol.
- On therapeutic basis
  - i. Those used for raising BP, e.g. noradrenaline.
  - ii. Those used as central stimulant, e.g. amphetamine.
  - iii. Those used as smooth muscle relaxants, e.g. adrenaline, salbutamol.
  - iv. Those used in allergic condition, e.g. adrenaline, ephedrine.
  - v. Those used for local vasoconstrictor effect, e.g. adrenaline, naphazoline.
  - vi. Those used for suppressing the appetite (anorexiants), e.g. phenfluramine, phenteramine.

Q 2. Name the receptors on which following drugs act.

1. Adrenaline acts on α- and β-receptors
2. Noradrenaline acts on α-receptors
3. Isoprenaline acts on β-receptors

Q 3. What are the effects of adrenergic receptor stimulation on different organs?

Adrenergic receptor	*Organ*	*Effect*
1. α-Receptors	Peripheral blood vessels	Vasoconstriction
	Eyes	Mydriasis
	Uterine smooth muscles	Constriction
	Intestinal smooth muscles	Contraction
2. β-Receptors	Heart	Increase contractility Increase heart rate
	Bronchi	Bronchodilation
	Skeletal blood vessels	Vasodilation
	Uterine smooth muscles	Relaxation
	Intestinal smooth muscles	Relaxation
	Liver	Glycogenolysis

Q 4. Give the pharmacological actions, adverse effects, therapeutic uses, preparations, contraindications of adrenaline (epinephrine).

Adrenaline (Epinephrine)

Pharmacological Actions

1. **On heart:** Adrenaline increases heart rate, force of contraction and cardiac output, i.e. it produces +ve and –ve chronotropic effect.
2. **Blood vessel and BP:** Adrenaline increases the BP due to its direct effect on heart and vasoconstriction of blood vessels.
3. **On smooth muscles:** Adrenaline relaxes the bronchial smooth muscles and produces bronchodilation. Adrenaline reduces GIT motility.
4. **On eye:** Adrenaline produces dilation of pupils, i.e. mydriasis.

Adverse Effects

1. Severe hypertension
2. Palpitation
3. Cardiac arrhythmia
4. Acute pulmonary edema
5. Fear, anxiety, restlessness
6. Headache, tremors

Therapeutic uses

1. In bronchial asthma
2. In allergic reactions
3. In cardiac arrest
4. To control the haemorrhage
5. It is added to local anaesthetic injections.

Preparation

Adrenaline injection (1:1000) IP 0.2–0.5 ml by SC/IM.

Contraindications

1. Hypertension
2. Thyrotoxicosis
3. Arteriosclerosis
4. Spinal anaesthesia.

Q 5. Explain 'Dale's vasomotor reversal' phenomenon.

Adrenaline is a mixed agonist which produces an increase in systolic but decrease in diastolic blood pressure.

A secondary fall occurs when the concentration of adrenaline decreases. The drugs like ergotoxin reverses the actions of adrenaline which is called "Dale's vasomotor reversal".

The vasoconstrictor action of adrenaline is blocked by ergot alkaloids. This may lead to stimulation of both receptors by adrenaline and thus causing a fall in blood pressure.

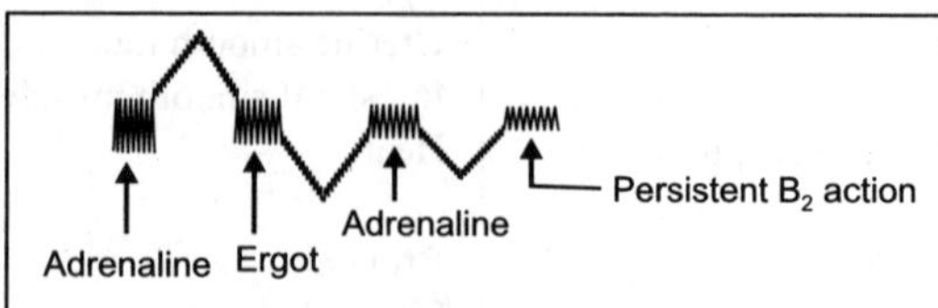

Dale's vasomotor reversal

The high dose of adrenaline with ergot extract also blocks the effects of adrenaline.

Q 6. Give the pharmacological actions, adverse effects, therapeutic uses, preparations of ephedrine.

Ephedrine

Ephedrine is alkaloid obtained from Ephedra plant.

Pharmacological Actions

1. **On CVS:** Ephedrine increases force of contraction of heart which result in increased cardiac output. It causes peripheral vasoconstriction hence blood pressure increases.
2. **On smooth muscles:** It produces relaxation of bronchial smooth muscles and also uterine smooth muscles.
3. **On CNS:** Ephedrine stimulates CNS and produces restlessness, insomnia, tremors and increased mental activity. In large doses may produce convulsions.
4. **On eye:** It produces mydriasis.
5. **Metabolic effect:** Ephedrine increases the metabolic rate of oxygen consumption.

Adverse Effects

1. Palpitation
2. Tachycardia
3. Headache, confusion, agitation
4. Insomnia
5. Emotional disturbances
6. Habituation, tolerance, dependance
7. Delirium, suicidal tendencies after larger dose.

Therapeutic uses

1. In bronchial asthma
2. As a nasal decongestant
3. In heart block
4. As a mydriatic
5. In narcolepsy
6. In whooping cough
7. In dysmenorrhoea
8. In hypotension during spinal anaesthesia

Contraindications

Ephedrine is contraindicated in:

- Closed angle glaucoma
- Hypertension
- Angina pectoris
- Cardiac arrhythmia.

Dosage

- Ephedrine tablet : 15–60 mg daily
- Ephedrine HCl syrup : 20 mg/ml
- Ephedrine nasal drops : 1%
- Ephedrine eye drops : 3 to 5%

Brand name: Medihaler Epi.

Q 7. Give the pharmacological actions, adverse effects, therapeutic uses, brand names of amphetamine.

Amphetamine

Pharmacological Actions

1. **Cardiovascular system:** It elevates the blood pressure systematically and diastolically. The cardiac effect is varying. Hpertensive action tachyphylaxis is generated.
2. **Central nervous system:** It is like caffeine, a strong CNS stimulant. It causes wakefulness at therapeutic dosages, postpones weariness and enhances physical performance. Mental and physical activity is increased. It could lead to euphoria, unrest, shivering, bewilderment and headaches. Fatigue and depression frequently follow repeated and excessive activation of the medication.
3. **Smooth muscles:** Only in large doses it relaxes smooth muscle of bronchi.
4. **Appetite suppressant:** It reduces appetite probably by acting on hypothalamic area concerned with feeding.
5. **Miscellaneous:** It has moderate anticonvulsant activity and is useful in petit mal epilepsy.

Adverse Effects

- Palpitation
- Confusion
- Calmness
- Restlessness
- Headache
- Habituation
- Tolerance

Therapeutic uses

Amphetamine is mainly used for its central effects:
1. Narcolepsy
2. As an anorexiant (reduces appetite) to reduce food intake in obese people.

Dosage

- Amphetamine tablet : 5–10 mg t.i.d orally

Brand name: Benzedrine.

Q 8. Give the uses, dose, route, adverse effects brand names of following adrenergic drugs.

Adrenergic Drugs

Drug	*Brand name*	*Dose*	*Route*	*Major adverse effect*
1. Adrenaline	Medicreme	1:1000 aqueous solution	IM/SC	Palpitation, hypertension
2. Isoprenaline	Isoproterenol, Isoprin	1–2 mg daily	Sublingual/ IM	Palpitation, tachycardia
3. Dopamine	Intropine	0.2 to 1 mg/min	IV infusion	Tachycardia, ectopic beats
4. Ephedrine	Medihaler Epi	05–3% 15–50 mg	Topical IV/ IM/SC	Palipitation, severe hypotension
5. Amphetamine	Benzedrine	5–10 mg twice daily	Oral	Palpitation, tremors

D. ANTIADRENERGICS

Q 1. Define and classify antiadrenergic drugs with examples.

Antiadrenergics

The drugs which block the actions produced by stimulation of sympathetic nervous system are called antiadrenergics.

These are also known as sympatholytics/adrenergic antagonists/adrenergic blockers.

Classification

1. α-Adrenergic blockers (α-blockers), e.g. phentolamine, tolazoline, ergot alkaloids, phenoxybenzamine.
2. β-Adrenergic blockers (β-blockers), e.g. propranolol, metoprolol, labetalol.
3. Adrenergic neuron blockers, e.g. guanethidine, bretylium.

According to mechanism of action of antiadrenergics is classified as:

a. Catecholamine depletor, e.g. reserpine.
b. Drugs that interfere with synthesis of adrenergic transmitters, e.g. α-methyldopa.
c. Drugs interfering with the transmission of impulses across post-ganglionic neurone, e.g. guanethidine.

Q 2. Write a note on α-adrenergic blockers.

α-Adrenergic Blockers

The drugs which block/antagonise the α-adrenergic receptor effects of adrenaline and noradrenaline are called α-adrenergic blockers.

Classification

1. β-Haloalkyl amines, e.g. dibenamine, phenoxybenzamine.
2. Natural and dihydrogenated ergot alkaloids, e.g. ergotoxine.
3. Imidazoline derivatives, e.g. tolazoline, phentolamine.
4. Miscellaneous, e.g. dibenzazepine, chlorpromazine.

Mechanism of Action

- α-Adrenergic receptor blockers selectively block the adrenergic responses by acting on effector organs, i.e. post-synaptically to block specific adrenergic receptors.
- The most prominent action of α-blocker is reduction in blood pressure and this action is due to peripheral vasodilation.
- α-Adrenergic receptor blockers may be reversible or irreversible.
- Reversible blockers dissociate from the receptors so that their effects may persist long after the drug has been cleared from the plasma, e.g. phenoxybenzamine.

Therapeutic uses/Indications of α-Adrenergic Blockers

1. Phentolamine is used in treatment of pheochromocytoma.
2. Tolazoline is used in Raynaud's disease, thrombophlebitis, etc.
3. Ergotamine is used in treatment of migraine.
4. Phenoxybenzamine is used in the treatment of pheochromocytoma.

Q 3. Write a note on β-adrenergic blockers.

β-Blockers

The drugs which block the actions on β-receptor are called β-blockers.

Classification

1. Specific β-blockers, e.g. sotalol, timolol.
2. β-Blockers with membrane stabilizing activity and intrinsic sympathomimetic activity, e.g. dichloroisoprenaline (DCI).
3. β-Blockers with membrane stabilizing activity, e.g. propranolol.
4. β-Blockers with additional β-blocking activity, e.g. labetalol.

Adverse Effects

1. Bradycardia
2. Sudden hypotension
3. Heart failure
4. Nausea, vomiting
5. Bronchospasm
6. Mental depression
7. Cold extremities, absent pulses

Therapeutic uses

1. In angina pectoris
2. In myocardial infarction
3. In cardiac arrhythmias
4. In hypertension
5. In thyrotoxicosis

Preparations

- Propranolol : 20 mg–2 mg daily in divided doses : Inderal
- Metaprolol : 150–300 mg once daily : Lopressor
- Labetalol : 80–400 mg twice daily : Normadate
- Pindolol : 1–45 mg daily : Visken
- Atenolol : 50–100 mg daily : Aten

Pharmacological Actions

1. β-Blockade Effect

These drugs do not cause any marked effect on normal heat. In case of increased sympathetic tone, the β-blockade in heart prevents increase in heart rate, cardiac output and myocardial contractility. These drugs reduce myocardial oxygen requirements and improve exercise tolerance in patients with angina. β-Blockers also reduce blood pressure by their action on heart and reduction in cardiac output. β-receptor blockade in bronchi may produce increased airway resistance which could be dangerous in patients with asthma.

2. Membrane Stabilizing Action

Propranolol has direct depressant effect on heart. This effect occurs only at higher doses. Because of this effect, myocardial contractility is depressed.

3. Intrinsic Sympathomimetic Activity

Some of β-blockers possess β-receptor stimulating activity (partial agonist property). Thus, though dichloroisoproterenol (DCI) blocks effect of adrenaline on heart, bronchi and blood vessels in absence of catecholamines. It increases heart rate, lowers blood pressure and causes increase in blood sugar.

4. Central Nervous System

Propranolol is capable of crossing blood–brain barrier due to high lipid solubility. As a result of this, it alters the mood of person.

Q 4. Write a note on 'propranolol'.

Propranolol

Propranolol is a non-selective β-adrenergic blocker.

Pharmacological Actions

The propranolol produces the following pharmacological actions:

1. *On cardiovascular system*
   - Bradycardia • Reduces blood pressure • Reduces force of contraction
2. *On respiratory system*
   - Bronchoconstriction, Metabolic system • Hypoglycemia
3. *On central nervous system*
   - Anti-anxiety action
4. *On eye*
   - Decrease the rate of aqueous humor production
5. *On kidneys*
   - Decrease renin secretion
6. *On metabolic system*
   - Hypoglycemia

Indications/Therapeutic uses

a. Cardiac arrhythmias
b. Hypertension
c. Prophylaxis against angina
d. Myocardial infarction
e. Thyrotoxicosis
f. Anxiety states
g. Prophylaxis against migraine attacks
h. Glaucoma

Adverse Reactions

- GI disturbances like nausea, vomiting
- Heart failure
- Heart block
- Hypotension and severe bradycardia
- Bronchospasm
- Allergic reaction
- Vivid dreams, night mare and hallucinations
- Cold hands
- Withdrawal symptoms in case of abrupt discontinuation
- Masking of hypoglycemia in diabetic patients

Contraindications

1. Bronchial asthma
2. Diabetes mellitus
3. Heart failure
4. Peripheral vascular disease

Q 5. Give the uses, doses, route, adverse effects, brand names of the following antiadrenergic drugs.

Antiadrenergics

Drug	*Brand name*	*Dose*	*Route*	*Major adverse effect*
1. Phenoxybenzamine	Dibenzyline	20–60 mg daily	Oral	Nasal congestion, miosis
2. Ergotoxine	Ergotox	0.5 mg twice daily	Oral, IV slowly	Myocardial infarction
3. Tolazoline	Prescoline	20–50 mg twice daily	Oral	Tachycardia
4. Phentolamine	Regitine	50 mg 4–6 times daily	Oral	Tachycardia
5. Sotalol	Betacardone, Sotagard	80 mg daily in divided doses	Oral	Ventricular arrhythmia
6. Timolol	Blocarden, Timolo	0.25–0.5% one drop twice daily	Topical	Ocular irritation
7. Propranolol	Inderal	10–40 mg twice daily	Oral	Hypotension, bradycardia
8. Labetalol	L-Beta	50 twice daily	Oral	Nasal stiffness, dyspepsia

E. NEUROMUSCULAR BLOCKING AGENTS

Q 1. What are neuromuscular blocking agents/neuromuscular blockers? Classify with examples.

Neuromuscular Blocking Agents

The drugs which block neuromuscular transmission at the neuromuscular junction, causing paralysis of the affected skeletal muscles are called neuromuscular blocking agents.

Classification of Neuromuscular Blocking Agents

1. **Depolarizing blockers:** For example succinylcholine (suxamethonium), decamethonium.

2. **Non-depolarizing blockers:** These are further classified on the basis of duration of action.
   a. ***Long acting:*** For example d-tubocurarine, pancuronium, poxacurium, pipecuronium.
   b. ***Intermediate acting:*** For example vecuronium, atricurium, rapacuronium, alcuronium.
   c. ***Short acting:*** For example miracurium.

Mechanism of Action

The nicotinic acetylcholine receptors exist at neuromuscular junction and ganglia and several pharmacological agents act at these receptors. The neuromuscular blocking agents depolarisation of motor end plate causing interference in neuromuscular transmission at neuromuscular junction. This results into relaxation of skeletal muscles or even paralysis of skeletal muscles.

Examples

1. **Succinylcholine:** It physically resemble acetylcholine and acts as an acetylcholine receptor agonist. It is not metabolized locally at neuromuscular junction, but metabolized by pseudocholinesterase in plasma. The continuous end plate depolarization causes muscle relaxation. It is mainly used to facilitate intubation. The onset is quick and duration of action is about 10 minutes.
2. **d-tubocurarine:**

- d-tubocurarine is an active ingredient of curare, an arrow poison.
- It works by binding to and blocking the nicotinic acetylcholine receptors of skeletal muscles at the neuromuscular junction.
- It was used in conjunction with an anaesthetic to provide skeletal muscle relaxation during surgery.

F. DRUGS USED IN MYASTHENIA GRAVIS

Q 1. What is myasthenia gravis? Give its treatments.

Myasthenia gravis: It is a chronic disease characterised by abnormal skeletal muscle weakness and fatigability.

It is now considered as autoimmune disease caused by the deficiency of the postsynaptic neuromuscular acetylcholine receptor complex.

Signs and Symptoms

1. Weakness of muscles of eye
2. Diplopia
3. Difficulty in chewing, swallowing
4. Slurring of speech
5. Respiratory failure due to weakness of respiratory muscles.

Drugs of Choice

Neostigmine, physostigmine, pyridostigmine.

Treatment

- Anticholinesterases act by inhibiting acetylcholinesterase, thereby prolonging the action of acetylcholine and thus enhancing neuromuscular transmission.
- *Neostigmine*:
  a. Neostigmine bromide 15 mg tablets are used.
  b. When injection is required neostigmine methylsulfate 500 μg/ml of 2.5 mg/ml are used.
  c. In myasthenic crisis, the intramuscular or subcutaneous injection of neostigmine is usually preferred.
- *Pyridostigmine*: It has slower onset but longer duration of effect than neostigmine and cause fewer muscarinic effects such as salivation, diarrhoea, abdominal cramps, hence usually preferred. Pyridostigmine bromide tablet 60 mg and injection 1 mg/ml are available.
- Glucocorticoids have shown clinical improvement in many myasthenia gravis patients.
- In some cases immunosuppressive agents like corticosteroids shown improvement in myasthenia gravis patients.

QUESTIONS: GIVE THE REASONS

Q 1. Why is acetylcholine not given/used clinically? Or Why the action of acetylcholine is very short lived? Or Why acetylcholine has a short duration of action?

i. It is a quaternary ammonium compound and is not effective orally.
ii. Acetylcholine is hygroscopic in nature.
iii. It is rapidly hydrolysed into acetic acid and choline.
iv. Acetylcholine is not used clinically because it acts on all cholinergic sites throughout the body.
v. Acetylcholine has short duration of action because it is susceptible to hydrolysis by cholinesterase.

$$\text{ACh} + \text{Ch E} \rightleftharpoons \underset{\text{Acetylated cholinesterase}}{\text{ACh Ch E}} \rightarrow \text{Ac Ch E} + \text{Choline} \xrightarrow{H_2O} \underset{\text{Regenerated cholinesterase}}{\text{Ch E}} + \text{Acetic acid}$$

vi. ACh when given orally, it is rapidly hydrolysed in GIT.
vii. On intravenous administration, it has no appreciable actions because considerable amount of ACh is destroyed by pseudocholinesterase in plasma and by true cholinesterase at the site of action. Thus, ACh has very short (transient) duration of action.

viii. ACh does not cross blood–brain barrier and hence does not exert any significant central action. Therefore, ACh is not used clinically.

Q 2. Why is adrenaline inactive orally?

i. On oral administration, adrenaline is rapidly inactivated in GIT by catechol orthomethyl transferase (COMT) and monoamine oxidase (MAO) enzymes.
ii. Also adrenaline is excreted immediately when given orally.

Hence, adrenaline is not administered orally.

Q 3. Why is adrenaline never administered intravenously?

i. Adrenaline has direct action on peripheral, skeletal blood vessels and heart.
ii. If adrenaline is administered intravenously it may increase sudden blood levels which is to be toxic.
iii. It may also produce palpitation, severe hypertension, arrhythmia in larger doses.

Hence, adrenaline is never administered intravenously.

Q 4. Why is adrenaline/salbutamol used in bronchial asthma?

i. In bronchial asthma, there is a bronchoconstriction and abnormal breathing.
ii. Adrenaline is a bronchodilator and immediately produces dilation of bronchi and relaxation of bronchial smooth muscles and improves breathing.
iii. Adrenaline inhibits mucosal secretions.

Hence, adrenaline is used in bronchial asthma.

Q 5. Why atropine produces photophobia?

i. The cholinergic nerves are supplied to circular muscles of iris which causes constriction of pupil.
ii. But atropine blocks the cholinergic nerve supply and causes dilation of pupil (mydriasis).
iii. Atropine paralyse the ciliary smooth muscles causing increase in the focal length of the lens. Thus, individual can see the things only at long distance.
iv. As muscles of sphincter of iris are paralysed, individual cannot constrict the pupil for viewing near objects or in response to bright light. Thus, atropine produces photophobia.

Q 6. Why adrenaline is always present in the emergency kit of physician?

It is because the adrenaline is a life saving drug. It is the drug of choice in the following clinical conditions:

i. **Anaphylatic shock:** Adrenaline acts as competitive antagonist of histamine. Anaphylactic shock is due to release of histamine which causes bronchospasm.

ii. **Cardiac shock (hypotensive):** As it is positive inotropic and positive chronotropic agent, it increases BP.

iii. **Asthma:** The bronchodilator action of adrenaline relieves the asthma due to bronchospasm.

iv. **Haemostatic:** The peripheral vasoconstrictor property of adrenaline is used to stop nasal and dental bleeding by using nasal or dental packs soaked in adrenaline solution.

v. **Adrenaline:** It is frequently administered along with local anaesthetic agent to prolong the duration of anaesthesia.

Q 7. Why is tincture of belladonna (atropine) used in diarrhoea?

i. Tincture of belladonna contains atropine which causes decrease in tone and motility (peristalsis) and produces constipation.

ii. In diarrhoea condition, there is an increased motility and evacuation of watery stools.

Q 8. Why adrenaline is used in the treatment of epistaxis (nose bleeding), why? OR Why are packs soaked in adrenaline preferred in dental practice after tooth extraction?

i. Adrenaline is a peripheral vasoconstrictor.

ii. When adrenaline is used as haemostatic agent, it produces vasoconstriction which stops bleeding.

Q 9. Why is atropine used in peptic ulcer?

i. Hypersecretion of HCl is one of the causes of peptic ulcer.

ii. In peptic ulcer, there is a hypersecretion of gastric juice.

iii. Atropine is an antisecretory agent and thus blocks all exocrine secretions.

iv. Hence, atropine assists ulcer-healing process.

Q 10. In treatment of myasthenia gravis, atropine is given along with neostigmine. Why?

i. Myasthenia gravis is a skeletal muscle disorder causing muscle weakness and muscle fatigue.

ii. Nicotinic receptors are present in skeletal muscles.

iii. Neostigmine being a parasympathomimetic (cholinergic) drug acts on both muscarinic and nicotinic receptors.

iv. Muscarinic receptors are present in heart, blood vessels and eyeballs.

v. In myasthenia gravis, only nicotinic action of neostigmine is required. Hence, to mask the muscarinic actions of neostigmine, the muscarinic blocker atropine is given along with neostigmine.

Q 11. Why edrophonium is used in the diagnosis of myasthenia gravis?

i. Edrophonium is structurally related to neostigmine having weak anti-cholinesterase activity.
ii. Edrophonium acts on skeletal muscles in too low doses.
iii. The duration of action of edrophonium is much shorter than neostigmine.
iv. The muscarinic effects of edrophonium are less prominent or negligible which can easily be countered by atropine.
v. A single dose of neostigmine (1 mg IM injection) used for diagnosis of myasthenia gravis produces marked improvement in muscle power which remains for 3–4 hours while edrophonium (10 mg IV injection) the effect remains only for 10 minutes.
Therefore, edrophonium is used in diagnosis of myasthenia gravis.

Q 12. Why ephedrine is preferred to atropine to produce mydriasis in elderly patients?

i. Ephedrine interacts with α-adrenergic receptors in the eye and produces mydriasis without causing cycloplegia and photophobia.
ii. Atropine produces mydriasis by causing paralysis of sphincter (circular) muscles of iris.
iii. Atropine also causes paralysis of ciliary smooth muscles and tightening of suspensory ligaments.
iv. This effect of atropine results in cycloplegia and photophobia which lasts for 1–10 days.
v. To avoid such visual complications, ephedrine is preferred to atropine to produce mydriasis in elderly patients.

Q 13. Neostigmine is the drug of choice in myasthenia gravis. Why?

i. Neostigmine being the parasympathomimetic (cholinergic agent) it acts on nicotinic receptor of skeletal muscle and improves muscle power in myasthenic patient.
ii. Neostigmine being choline esterase inhibitor blocks and true pseudo-cholinesterase and sets free acetylcholine which in turn acts on nicotinic receptor of skeletal muscle and improves muscle power.
iii. Thus, in a single therapeutic dose, neostigmine produces marked striking improvement in muscle power in myasthenic, individuals.

Objective Questions with Answers in Bold Letters

1. **Acetylcholine** is a neurotransmitter of parasympathetic nervous system (PNS).
2. Adrenaline/noradrenaline/dopamine are neurotransmitters of **sympathetic nervous system** (SNS).
3. **Pilocarpine** is a cholinomimetic alkaloid.

4. Adrenaline is also known as **epinephrine**.
5. **Ephedrine** is an alkaloid obtained from Ephedra plant.
6. Phentolamine is used in the treatment of **pheochromocytoma**.
7. **Propranolol** is a β-adrenergic blocking agent.
8. Succinylcholine is an example of **depolarizing blockers**.
9. Neostigmine is a drug of choice in treatment of **myasthenia gravis**.
10. The neurotransmitter **acetylcholine** is a choline ester.
11. **Physostigmine** is used in the treatment of morphine poisoning.
12. **Pralidoxime (2–PAM)** is used in organophosphorus compound poisoning.
13. **Atropine** is an alkaloid obtained from *Atropa belladonna*.
14. **α-Receptors** are found in the autonomic ganglia, skeletal muscles and adrenal medulla.
15. The cholinergic drugs are also called **cholinomimetics**.
16. Cholinergic blocking agents are also called **parasympatholytics**.
17. Atropine produce **mydriasis**.
18. Noradrenaline acts on **α-receptor**.
19. Isoprenaline acts on **β-receptor**.
20. **Acetylcholine** produce muscarinic and nicotinic actions.
21. **Atropine** reduces all exocrine secretions.
22. Atropine is a competitive antagonist of **acetylcholine**.
23. The drugs which supress appetite are called **anorexiants**.
24. **Ephedrine** is used in narcolepsy.
25. Atropine produces **photophobia**.
26. **Adrenaline** contains catechol nucleus.
27. Adrenaline acts on **α- and β-receptors**.
28. 'Dales vasomotor reversal phenomenon' is produced by **adrenaline and ergot**.
29. **Ephedrine** is a competitive inhibitor of MAO.
30. **Isoprenaline** is given by sublingual route in treatment of bronchial asthma.
31. Adrenergic antagonists are also known as **sympatholytics**.
32. Phenoxybenzamine is a **α-blocker**.
33. **Guanethidine** is an adrenergic neuron blocker.
34. **Reserpine** is a catecholamine depletor.
35. **Tolazoline** is used in treatment of Raynaud's disease.
36. Ergotamine is used in the treatment of **migraine**.
37. **Inderal** is a popular brand name of propranolol.
38. **Propranolol** is a non-selective β-adrenergic blocker.
39. **d-tubocurarine** is a long acting neuromuscular blocking agent.
40. **Adrenaline** is used in bronchial asthma.
41. **Atropine** is used in peptic ulcer.
42. **Adrenaline** is always present in the emergency kit of the physician.

43. Edrophonium is used in the diagnosis of **myasthenia gravis**.
44. In the treatment myasthenia gravis, atropine is given along with **neostigmine**.
45. Phenoxybenazamine is used in the treatment of **Raynaud's disease**.
46. **Pilocarpine** is used in an **open angle glaucoma**.
47. Acetylcholine produces **miosis**.
48. **Atropine** reduces tone, motility or peristalsis of GIT.
49. **Cycloplegia** means paralysis of accomodation.
50. The person fails to respond to bright light, this is known as **'photophobia'**.

G. LOCAL ANAESTHETIC AGENTS

Q 1. Define and classify local anaesthetics with examples. State the qualities of an ideal local anaesthetic.

Local Anaesthetics

The drugs which produce anaesthesia is limited/localised area of the body are called local anaesthetics.

Classification

1. **Ester Type:**
   a. Benzoic acid ester, e.g. cocaine, amylocaine.
   b. Para-aminobenzoic acid ester, e.g. procaine, amethocaine, benzocaine, orthocaine.
2. **Amide Type:**
   a. Acetanilide derivatives, e.g. xylocaine (lidocaine).
   b. Quinoline derivatives, e.g. cinchocaine.

The Properties of an Ideal Local Anaesthetic

i. It should be nonirritating to the tissue.
ii. It should be stable in water and lipid.
iii. It should have quick onset of action and sufficient duration of action.
iv. It should not cause permanent damage to nerves.
v. It should not have any little systemic toxicity.
vi. It should be stable, easily sterilizable and inexpensive and should be safe.
vii. It should be cheap and easily available.

Q 2. Give the mechanism of action of local anaesthetics.

Local anaesthetics block both the generation and conduction of nerve impulses. The blockade results from biochemical changes caused by the drug on the lipotrophic film of cell membrane.

The lipophillic activity is essential for migration of drug into the neuronal fibre while water solubility is essential to get the drug to the site of action from site of injection or application.

Q 3. What are different methods/ways of producing local anaesthesia?

Local anaesthesia can be produced by the following ways:

i. Drugs Acting by Paralysing Sensory Nerve Ending

- By application to the mucous surface, e.g. cocaine, cinchocaine, amethocaine.
- By hypodermic injection, e.g. procaine–2%, amithocaine 0.1%, cinchocaine 0.05%.
- By infiltration.
- By application to wounds.
- By application to the skin.

ii. Drugs Blocking the Sensory Impulse

- *Block anaesthesia:* Procaine is injected close to the nerve trunk.
- *Spinal anaesthesia:* Procaine, amylocaine. Drug is introduced after lumbar puncture.
- *By producing caudal anaesthesia:* Procaine is injected into the epidural space.

Q 4. Give the adverse effects, therapeutic uses, brand names of lignocaine/xylocaine.

Lignocaine

- It is a commonly used local anaesthetic and is most stable.
- It has quick onset of action and high degree of penetration.
- It is a potent local anaesthetic agent.

Adverse Effects

i. Hypotension
ii. Bradycardia
iii. Convulsions
iv. Respiratory paralysis
v. Skin sensitization
vi. Allergic dematitis
vii. A typical asthmatic attack.

Therapeutic uses

i. It is used for topical anaesthesia
ii. For infiltration anaesthesia
iii. For nerve block anaesthesia
iv. For spinal anaesthesia
v. For dental anaesthesia
vi. As an antiarrhythmic agent.

Trade Names: Xylocaine, Xylocard, Lidocaine.

Q 5. Give the uses, dose, brand names, route, adverse effects of following local anaesthetics.

Local Anaesthetics

Drug	*Brand name*	*Dose*	*Route*	*Major adverse effect*
1. Cocaine	–	5–10% solution	Topical	Mydriasis
2. Procaine	Novocaine	1–2% solution	Injection	Anaphylaxis, tachycardia
3. Lignocaine	Xylocaine, Xylocard, Gesicaine	20 mg/ml solution 4% solution	Injection Topical	Tachycardia Hypotension, mental clouding
4. Amethocaine	Anethane	0.25–0.5% solution	Topical and injection	Hypotension
5. Cinchocaine	Nupercaine, Nupercainal	0.5% solution	Injection	Hypotension

QUESTION: GIVE THE REASONS

Q 1. Why adrenaline is added to injections of local anaesthetics? OR Why adrenaline is given along with procaine to produce local anaesthesia?

i. Adrenaline is a sympathomimetic agent while procaine is local anaesthetic.
ii. Procaine is vasodilator drug while adrenaline causes vasoconstriction.
iii. When given in combination, adrenaline causes peripheral vasoconstriction.
iv. This results in decreased systemic absorption of procaine and prolonged duration of action.
v. The systemic toxicity of procaine is also reduced.
vi. Hence, adrenaline is given along with procaine to produce local anaesthesia.

Objective Questions with Answers in Bold Letters

1. **Local anaesthetics** are the drugs which produce anaesthesia in limited area of the body.
2. Lignocaine is an **amide type** of local anaesthetic.
3. **Cinchocaine** is a quinoline derivative used as local anaesthetic.
4. Local anaesthetics block the **generation and conduction of nerve impulses.**
5. In block anaesthesia procaine is injected close to the **nerve trunk.**
6. In **spinal anaesthesia** the drug is injected through lumbar puncture.
7. In caudal anaesthesia drug is injected in **epidural space.**
8. Cocaine produces **topical anaesthesia.**
9. Xylocaine is a popular brand name of **lignocaine.**
10. **Adrenaline** is added to injections of local anaesthetics.

H. NONSTEROIDAL ANTI-INFLAMMATORY DRUGS (NSAIDs)

Q 1. Define the terms.

1. **Analgesics:** The drugs which reduce pain sensation are called analgesics.
2. **Antipyretics:** The drugs which reduce elevated body temperature to normal level are called antipyretics.
3. **Anti-inflammatory agents:** The drugs which are used in the treatment of inflammation are called anti-inflammatory agents.
4. **Inflammation:** Inflammation is a response triggered by damage to living tissues. Inflammation is characterized by pain, edema and rarely fever.
5. **Narcotic analgesics/opioid analgesics:** The drugs which reduce pain sensation along with loss of consciousness and sleep are known as narcotic analgesics/opioid analgesics.
6. **Non-narcotic analgesics (plain analgesics):** These are the drugs which reduce pain sensation without inducing sleep and unconsciousness are called non-narcotic analgesics.
7. **Nonsteroidal anti-inflammatory drugs (NSAIDs):** The drugs which are used to reduce inflammatory and do not have steroid ring in their chemical structure are called nonsteroidal anti-inflammatory drugs (NSAIDs), e.g. aspirin, paracetamol, phenylbutazone, indomethacin, ibuprofen, diclofenac.

Q 2. Define and classify NSAIDs. OR Classify analgesic-antipyretic and anti-inflammatory drugs.

NSAIDs: The drugs which are used to reduce inflammation and do not contain steroidal ring in their chemical structure are called NSAIDs.

Classification of NSAIDs/Analgesic-antipyretics and Anti-inflammatory Drugs

1. Salicylates and their derivatives, e.g. aspirin, sodium salicylate.
2. p-aminophenol derivatives, e.g. paracetamol, phenacetin.
3. Pyrazolone derivatives, e.g. phenylbutazone, oxyphenbutazone.
4. Indole-acetic acid derivatives, e.g. indomethacin, sulindac.
5. Phenylacetic acid derivatives, e.g. diclofenac.
6. Propionic acid derivatives, e.g. ibuprofen, ketoprofen, fenoprofen.
7. Fenamates, e.g. mefenamic acid, fluphenamic acid.
8. Oxicams, e.g. piroxicam.

Q 3. Write a noe on salicylates (aspirin).

Aspirin (Salicylates)

- The salicylates are the esters or salts of salicylic acid.
- Salicylates are always given orally.

- Salicylates are the most widely used and effective analgesics.
- Aspirin is most extensively used.
- Aspirin is known as acetyl salicylic acid (ASA).

Absorption, Fate and Excretion (Pharmacokinetic)

- The stomach and small intestine absorb salicylates well.
- The absorption of salicylates is aided by the pH of stomach.
- To avoid gastrointestinal discomfort, salicylates are always given with food.
- Sodium bicarbonate is given along with salicylate/aspirin to avoid GIT discomfort.
- In the plasma and liver, aspirin is promptly deacetylated to create salicylic acid, which is subsequently conjugated by the liver and eliminated in the urine.

Pharmacological Actions of Salicylates (Aspirin)

I. *On CNS*

a. **Analgesic action:** Salicylates produce relief of pain without producing hypnosis or marked impairment in mental activity. Salicylates relieve pains by central as well as peripheral action.

b. **Antipyretic action:** Salicylates reduce excessive body temperature to the normal level by heat loss through sweating and vasodilation. In fever condition, prostaglandin substance is increased. The salicylates inhibit prostaglandin synthesis in the brain and lowers the body temperature.

c. **Anti-inflammatory action:** Salicylates reduce only the inflammatory component of disease without affecting tissue component. Salicylates reduce the capillary permeability by minimising the exudation of fluid and development of inflammatory edema. The salicylates inhibit the synthesis of prostaglandins and help to prevent pain and inflammation.

II. *Effect on Respiration*

Salicylates stimulate respiration as a result of direct and indirect actions.

III. *On GIT*

The acid pH of stomach leads to unionized form of salicylates. This nonionized form of salicylate is water insoluble hence it sticks to gastric mucosa and produces gastric irritation. To avoid gastric irritation, salicylates may be administered after food. Excessive use of salicylates may cause nausea, vomiting, epigastric distress, peptic ulceration, GIT haemorrhage, etc.

IV. *Antirheumatic Effect*

Salicylates have powerful anti-inflammatory action and are prostaglandin inhibitors thus help to prevent pain and inflammation associated with rheumatism.

V. *Antigout Action/Uricosuric Effect*

When salicylates are administered in the dose of more than 5 gm/ day, it prevents reabsorption of uric acid and increases its excretion. Hence, due to uricosuric property they are used in gout.

VI. *Local Action*

Methyl salicylate produces counterirritant and rubefacient action.

Adverse Effects/Toxic Effects of Salicylates

1. **Allergic reactions:** Skin rash, urticaria, bronchial asthma.
2. **GIT toxicity:** GIT irritation, nausea, vomiting, GIT bleeding, hyperpyrexia, convulsions, epigastric pains, coma, dehydration, deafness, respiratory alkalosis.
3. **Salicylism:** Prolonged administration of salicylates produces a mild salicylate intoxication termed salicylism. Salicylism is characterised by headache, deafness, mental confusion, vomiting, diarrhoea.
4. Hypoprothrombinemia.

Therapeutic uses of Salicylates (Aspirin)

1. As analgesic and antipyretic.
2. As anti-inflammatory agents.
3. In the treatment of rheumatic fever and rheumatoid arthritis.
4. Aspirin has been used to prevent the formation of platelet fibrin thrombus.
5. Salicylic acid also has keratolytic, fungistatic, mild antiseptic activity.
6. Methyl salicylate is used as counterirritant and rubefacient.

Preparation: Aspirin tablet IP

Dose: 4–8 gm daily in divided doses.

Trade Names: Aspro, Disprin.

Contraindications

Aspirin/salicylates are contraindicated in:

- Hypersensitivity (urticaria, angioedema, asthma)
- Peptic ulcer (gastrointestinal ulceration)
- Haemophilia
- Bleeding disorders.

Q 4. Define anti-inflammatory drugs. Give therapeutic uses of anti-inflammatory drugs.

Anti-inflammatory Drugs

The drugs which are used to reduce inflammation are called anti-inflammatory drugs.

Therapeutic uses of Anti-inflammatory Drugs

i. Headache
ii. Rheumatoid arthritis
iii. Rheumatism
iv. Toothache
v. Migraine
vi. Arthritis
vii. Ankylosing spondylitis
viii. Antigout

Q 5. Write a note on 'acute salicylate poisoning.

Acute Salicylate Poisoning (Salicylism)

A larger dose of salicylate can cause salicylate poisoning.

Symptoms

1. Deep and rapid breathing (hypercapnea).
2. Anorexia
3. Nausea, vomiting, thirst, diarrhoea.
4. Headache, dizziness, deafness, dimness of vision.
5. Confusion, restlessness, disorientation, delirium, mania, hallucination.
6. Deep coma, respiratory and circulatory collapse.
7. High fever
8. GIT bleeding, epigastric pains, GIT irritation.

Treatment

1. Gastric lavage is done with water or sodium bicarbonate (3.5%).
2. Administration of milk or slurry of universal antidote.
3. Saline cathartics like sodium sulphate or magnesium sulphate are used.
4. Checking of acid–base status of the patient.
5. Sodium bicarbonate is given by IV as an antidote.
6. To correct dehydration glucose saline is given.
7. Smaller doses of barbiturates, paraldehyde may be required to suppress the restlessness and convulsions.
8. For hyperpyrexia, use sponge bath.
9. For CNS depression, caffeine, nikethamide may be useful.

Q 6. Give the uses, doses, route, brand names, adverse effects of following anti-inflammatory drugs.

Analgesics, Anti-pyretics, Anti-inflammatory Drugs/Non-narcotics

Drug	*Brand name*	*Dose*	*Route*	*Major adverse effect*
1. Aspirin	Disprin, Actifed	300–600 mg daily	Oral	Heart-burn, methaemoglobinemia
2. Paracetamol	Crocin, Calpol, Paramol, Febrex Plus	0.5–1 gm daily	Oral	Methaemoglobinemia, blood dyscrasias
3. Phenylbutazone	Butazolidine	400 mg daily in divided doses	Oral	Haematuria, blood dyscrasias
4. Oxyphenbutazone	Suganril	400 mg daily in divided doses	Oral	Peptic ulcer, blood dyscrasias
5. Analgin	Baralgan, Novalgin	0.5 to 1 gm daily	Oral	
6. Indomethacin	Indocap, Indocin	25 mg 2–3 times daily	Oral	Light headedness, gastric bleeding
7. Mefenamic acid	Meftal Forte	0.5 gm 3 times a day	Oral	Diarrhoea, anemia
8. Ibuprofen	Brufen	400 mg twice daily	Oral	Headache, dizziness

QUESTIONS: GIVE THE REASONS

Q 1. Why aspirin is not used in patients with peptic ulcer?/Why aspirin is contraindicated in patients with peptic ulcer?

i. Aspirin causes irritation of stomach, gastric erosion, gastritis, gastric ulcer and GI bleeding.
ii. It also causes decrease in prostagladin level leading to increased secretion of HCl.
iii. Aspirin stimulates the CTZ in the brain causing epigastric distress, nausea and vomiting. Hence, it is not used in patients with peptic ulcer.

Q 2. Why aspirin is generally taken after meal or in association with sodium bicarbonate?

i. If aspirin is taken on empty stomach, it causes gastric irritation, nausea and vomiting.
ii. It may also causes GI bleeding.
iii. Aspirin also increases the secretion of HCl in stomach, indirectly by decreasing prostaglandin level. This results in ulceration.
iv. Aspirin when administered after meal or with sodium bicarbonate, the acid secreted in the stomach gets neutralised by sodium bicarbonate. This avoids the gastric complications like GIT irritation, nausea, vomiting, etc.

Q 3. Why salicylate therapy is always supported with vitamin K?

i. Salicylates therapy can cause GI bleeding resulting in haematemesis and anemia.
ii. Salicylate in large doses reduces the plasma prothrombin level causing hypoprothrombinaemia.
iii. At low dose the disturbance in blood clotting is due to interference with prostaglandin synthesis.
iv. Hypoprothrombinaemia and haemorrhagic complications can be prevented or treated with stimultaneous administration of vitamin K.
v. Vitamin K favours coagulation, i.e. increases clotting and prevents GIT bleeding. Hence, vitamin K is supplemented with salicylates.

Q 4. Why is sodium bicarbonate given with aspirin or salicylate poisoning?

i. If aspirin is given alone, it sticks to the gastric mucosa due to unionized nature and causes gastric irritation.
ii. Sodium bicarbonate increases the ionization of salicylates and forms water-soluble sodium salicylates.

iii. Hence, administration of sodium bicarbonate increases the rate of excretion of aspirin and thus used as antidote in salicylate poisoning.

Objective Questions with Answers in Bold Letters

1. The drugs which reduce pain sensation are called **analgesics**.
2. The drugs which reduce elevated body temperature are called **antipyretics**.
3. The drugs which reduce inflammation are **anti-inflammatory** drugs.
4. **Paracetamol** is a para-aminophenol derivative.
5. **Sulindac** is an indole-acetic acid derivative.
6. Salicylates/aspirin is always given **orally**.
7. **Aspirin** is also known as acetylsalicylic acid (ASA).
8. **Sodium bicarbonate** is given along with salicylate/aspirin to avoid gastric discomfort.
9. Salicylates are **prostaglandin inhibitors**.
10. **Hypoprothombinemia** is a major toxic effect of salicylates/aspirin.
11. **Methyl salicylate** is used as counterirritant and rubefacient.
12. The dose of aspirin in an adult is **4–8 gm** daily in divided doses.
13. Aspirin is contraindicated in **peptic ulcer**.
14. Sodium bicarbonate is given by **IV** as an antidote in salicylate poisoning.
15. **Methaemoglobinemia** is an adverse effect of aspirin.
16. Disprin is a popular brand name of **aspirin**.
17. Aspirin is generally taken **after meals/on full stomach**.
18. Salicylate therapy is always supported with **vitamin K**.
19. **Sodium bicarbonate/alkali** is given in acute salicylate poisoning.
20. **Sulindac** is a strong **cyclooxygenase inhibitor**.
21. Ibuprofen is a potent inhibitor of **prostaglandin synthetase**.
22. **Diclofenac** is a phenylacetic acid derivative.

Chapter 3

Drugs Acting on Eye

- Miotics
- Drugs used in glaucoma
- Mydriatics

Q 1. What are miotics? Give the mechanism of action and therapeutic uses of miotics. OR 'Write a note on miotics'.

Miotics

The drugs which produce constriction of pupils are called miotics, e.g. acetylcholine, pilocarpine, carbachol, physostigmine.

Mechanism of Action

When miotics are instilled in eye, it causes contraction of circular muscle fibres and relaxation of radial muscle fibres.

This causes marked reduction in size of pupil which is referred as miosis. Because of miosis, focal length of pupil is also reduced. Thus, person can see the things which are near but fails to observe the things at long distance. This is known as paralysis of accommodation.

Therapeutic Applications

1. To treat glaucoma.
2. To break adhesion between iris and lens.
3. To control mydriasis and cycloplegia produced by atropine.

1. Pilocarpine

- Pilocarpine is a cholinergic agonists.
- It is a direct acting parasympathomimetic drug.
- Primarily it is used in the treatment of glaucoma.
- It is used in the form of eye drops solution.

Indications/Therapeutic uses

Pilocarpine is used in:

i. Chronic open-angle glaucoma
ii. Ocular hypertension
iii. In emergency treatment of acute angle-closure glaucoma.

Adverse Effects

- Eye pain
- Blurred vision
- Ciliary spasm
- Lacrimation
- Myopia

Contraindications

- Acute iritis
- Acute uveitis
- Inflammation of anterior segment

Dosage

i. Pilocarpine hydrochloride drops 2%, 4%.
ii. Pilocarpine nitrate drops 2%, 4% one drop up to four times daily.

Brand names: Pilocar, Opthocarpine, Salagen.

2. Timolol

It is a specific β-adrenergic blocker. It is combined with carbonic anhydrase inhibitor.

Indications/uses

Timolol is used in: a. Ocular hypertension, b. chromic open-angle glaucoma.

Contraindications

- Uncontrolled heart failure
- Bradycardia
- Heart block
- Asthma

Dosage

Timolol eye drops 0.25–0.5% twice daily.

Brand names: Blocarden, Timol

Q 2. What are mydriatics? Give mechanism of action, uses of mydriatics. OR Write a note on 'mydriatics'.

Mydriatics

The drugs which produce dilation of pupils are called mydriatics, e.g. adrenaline, ephedrine, cocaine, atropine, homatropine.

Mechanism of Action

When mydriatics are instilled in eye, it causes relaxation of circular muscle fibres and causes tightening of radial muscle fibres. This causes flattening of lens known as mydriasis.

Because of mydriasis, the focal length is also increased which fixes the sight for far vision, i.e. person can see the objects which are at long distance but fails to see the near objects. This is known as cycloplegia.

Therapeutic Applications

1. To produce mydriasis (mydriasis means dilation of pupils).
2. For ophthalmological examinations.

Atropine

- Anticholinergic drug, atropine by blocking muscarinic cholinergic effects, paralyse the pupillary constrictor muscle resulting into dilation of pupil (mydriasis).
- In addition, the paralysis of ciliary muscles result into paralysis of accommodation (cycloplegia).

Indications/Therapeutic uses

1. In iritis 2. In uveitis 3. Antispasmodic

Contraindications: Angle-closure glaucoma.

Dosage: Eumydrin.

Q 3. Write a note on 'glaucoma and its treatment'.

Glaucoma and its Treatment

Glaucoma is an ocular disease in which intraocular pressure is increased and causes damage to optic nerve producing visual loss.

The damage to optic nerve and visual loss is probably due to ischaemia (deficient blood supply to any part of the body) and may be due to direct pressure on nerve. Glaucoma is a major cause of blindness in persons over 40 years of age. There are two major types:

i. Open angle glaucoma, ii. narrow angle glaucoma.

Drugs used in Glaucoma

1. *Miotics:* Pilocarpine, carbachol, physostigmine.
2. *Adrenergic agents:* Adrenaline and pilocarpine mixture.
3. *β-Adrenergic blockers:* Timolol.
4. *Carbonic anhydrase inhibitor:* Acetazolamide.
5. Osmotic agents: Mannitol.
6. *Prostaglandin:* Latanoprost.
    1. **β-Adrenergic blockers:** Timolol, betaxolol and levobunolol are the β-blockers effective in glaucoma. They act by reducing the formation of aqueous humour.
    2. **Miotics:** Pilocarpine and physostigmine are the miotics used in glaucoma. They produce contraction of the ciliary muscle.
    3. **α-Adrenergic agonists:** The drugs used in apraclonidine and brimonidine. Both are congeners of clonidine. They act by decreasing aqueous humour production.

4. **Carbonic anhydrase inhibitors:** Acetazolamide belongs to this group. It acts by inhibiting the generation of bicarbonate ion in the ciliary epithelium.
5. **Prostaglandins:** Latanoprost is a drug used to treat increased pressure inside of the eye. It is a $PGF_{2\alpha}$ derivative. It can produce iris pigmentation and sometimes blurred vision. Latanoprost is applied as eye drops.

Objective Questions with Answers in Bold Letters

1. **Mydriatic agents** are known to produce mydriasis.
2. Mydriasis means **dilation of pupils**.
3. **Glaucoma** is a disease characterized by increase in intraocular tension.
4. **Miosis** means constriction of pupil.
5. **Timolol** is non-selective β-blocker that reduces the secretion of aqueous humour.
6. Pilocarpine is a **miotic** agent.
7. **Acetazolamide** is a carbonic anhydrase inhibitor and acts by reducing the production of aqueous humour in glaucoma.
8. In miosis, there is a marked **reduction in pupil size**.
9. **Pilocarpine** is a drug of choice in glaucoma.
10. **Mydriatics** causes relaxation of circular muscle fibres.
11. **Atropine** produces cycloplegia.

Chapter 4

Drugs Acting on Central Nervous System

- General anaesthetics
- Anticonvulsant drugs (antiepileptic drugs)
- Antidepressants/psychoanaleptics
- Nootropic agents
- Opioid analgesics
- Hypnotics and sedatives
- Antianxiety drugs/anxiolytics
- Antipsychotics
- Centrally acting muscle relaxants

A. GENERAL ANAESTHETICS

Q 1. What is anaesthesia? Explain various stages/mode of action/ mechanism of action of anaesthesia.

Anaesthesia

Anaesthesia is a state of controlled, temporary loss of sensation or awareness that is induced for medical purposes.

Stages of Anaesthesia (Mode/Mechanism of Anaesthesia)

a. Stage of Analgesia

This stage starts from beginning of inhalation of anaesthetic agent up to loss of consciousness. It involves sensation of falling, remoteness and feeling of warmth is observed in some patients. Analgesia is produced before consciousness is lost.

b. Stage of Delirium

This stage starts with loss of consciousness to beginning of surgical anaesthesia. This stage involves marked excitement, shouting, laughing, increased muscular activity, vomiting, pupils may dilate and patient shows development of marked hypertension and tachycardia.

c. Stage of Surgical Anaesthesia

As the more drug gets in, deep breathing starts and patient passes into the third stage. This gives gradual loss of reflexes, regular respiration and relaxation of skeletal muscle.

This stage is divided into four different planes:

Plane 1: The pupils are normal and eyeballs are roving. The pupils dilate and attain normal size. The respiration is full and regular. BP and pulse rate is normal.

Plane 2: Eyeballs are fixed and amplitude of respiration is diminished. Adequate muscular relaxation.

Plane 3: The BP begins to fall. Intercostal muscles are paralysed slowly. The pupillary light reflex is lost. Muscles relax completely.

Plane 4: Intercostal muscles completely paralysed. The pupils are further dilated. BP is low. All secretions are completely abolished.

d. Stage of Respiratory Paralysis

This stage is characterised by severe depression of vital medullary centres, initially the diaphragmic contractions are irregular. Respiratory arrest also leads to vasomotor collapse.

Four Planes of Surgical Anaesthesia

	Respiration	*Blood pressure*	*Reflex activity*	*Muscle relaxation*	*Pupils*
Plane 1	Full deep, thoracoabdominal decreased rate of respiration	Heart rate normal, blood pressure decreases	Loss of pharyngeal reflexes	Incomplete	Normal, roving eyeballs
Plane 2	Further decreased rate of respiration. Low amplitude of respiration	Heart rate normal, blood pressure further decreased	Laryngeal reflexes lost. Loss of skin incision reflex	Adequate	Fixed eyeballs. Eyelid reflex lost
Plane 3	Decreased rate of respiration. Respiration only abdominal	Hypotension	-do-	Complete	Dilated
Plane 4	Paralysis of respiration	Severe hypotension	-do-	Complete	More dilated

Q 2. Define and classify general anaesthetics giving examples.

General Anaesthetics

The drugs which produce a total or partial loss of the pain sensation along with loss of consciousness are called general anaesthetics.

Classification

1. Inhalation general anaesthetics
   a. **Volatile liquids:** For example, diethyl ether, chloroform, halothane, trichloroethylene, methoxy flurane, ethylchloride.
   b. **Gases:** For example, cyclopropane, nitrous oxide, ethylene.
2. Intravenous anaesthetics
   a. **Ultra short-acting barbiturates:** For example, thiopentone, methohexitone.
   b. **Nonbarbiturates:** For example, propandid, ketamine, althesin, etomidate.

Q 3. Write a note on 'volatile general anaesthetics'/inhalation anaesthetics.

Volatile General Anaesthetics

These are available in two forms.

a. **Liquids:** For example, diethyl ether, chloroform, halothane, methoxyflurane, ethylchloride, trichloroethylene.
b. **Gases:** Nitrous oxide, ethylene, cyclopropane.

1. Diethyl Ether (Anaesthetic Ether)

- Anaesthetic ether contains 96–98% diethyl ether.
- Ether is a colourless liquid of very volatile nature.
- Ether has characteristic odour, sweet burning taste.
- The concentration of 10–15% in inspired air is sufficient.

Pharmacological Action

- Only a minor portion of ether is oxidised in the body and is eliminated through the lungs.
- Ether irritates the respiratory tract and enhances the mucosal secretions.
- Ether is known to increase heart rate, blood pressure and blood sugar.
- Ether also causes peripheral vasodilation.
- Ether depresses myocardial contractility.

Adverse Effects

- Nausea, vomiting during recovery of anaesthesia.
- Very irritant and explosive anaesthetic.
- Children show a tendency to ether convulsions.

Contraindications

- Severe liver disease
- Impaired kidney function
- Diabetes mellitus

Therapeutic uses

- Safe general anaesthetic
- Used in pediatric anaesthesia
- Excellent analgesic
- Can be employed to reduce labour pains.

Dose: For induction of anaesthesia up to 15% in inspired air.

Advantages

1. It is a safe anaesthetic, can be used by unexperienced anaesthetist.
2. Preanaesthetic medication is not required.
3. It is an excellent analgesic.
4. Ether produces satisfactory muscular relaxation.

5. Ether does not modify blood pressure during anaesthetic stages.
6. Ether can be employed during delivery to reduce labour pains.
7. Ether can be administered without a complicated apparatus.
8. Ether anaesthesia is economical.

Disadvantages

1. Induction of anaesthesia is slow and is sometimes associated with marked excitement.
2. Irritant nature of the ether vapour may increase the salivary and bronchial secretions and induce cough and laryngeal spasms during induction of ether.
3. The heart rate is usually increases during ether anaesthesia.
4. Nausea and vomiting appear during recovery from ether anaesthesia.
5. The motility of GIT is reduced by ether and secretions are also depressed.

2. Chloroform

- It is a clear, volatile liquid of boiling point 61°C.
- It has a sweet, appreciable smell.
- In the presence of flame, it also decomposes to form phosgene.
- It is quickly absorbed and complete eliminated through lungs.

Pharmacological Actions

- It is a highly potent anaesthetic agent.
- It can produce all the stages of anaesthesia without causing hypoxia.
- Surgical anaesthesia can be achieved within 2 to 3 minutes.
- Chloroform produces arterial hypotension without much affecting the heart rate.
- Cardiac arrest may occur suddenly during chloroform administration.
- Chloroform gives a cooling sensation when dropped on the skin.
- Chloroform sometimes used as a rubefacient.

Adverse Effects

- Cirrhosis of liver
- Delayed chloroform poisoning
- Postanaesthetic toxemia
- Hypotension
- Cardiac arrest
- Arrhythmia
- Ventricular fibrillation and respiratory arrest
- Paralytic ileus.

Therapeutic uses

1. Chloroform is a powerful anaesthetic agent.
2. Chloroform is employed as counter-irritant and rubefacient.

3. Dilute solutions of chloroform administered internally as carminative, stomachic and flavouring agents.
4. Chloroform is used as a vehicle for extraction of organic drugs.

Advantages

1. It is a highly potent anaesthetic agent.
2. In very low concentration it acts as an analgesic.
3. Surgical anaesthesia can be achieved within 2–3 minutes.

Disadvantages

Chloroform is not a safe anaesthetic agent due to following toxic effects:

1. Chloroform depresses the respiratory centre.
2. It may produce arterial hypotension.
3. It may cause cardiotoxicity, hepatotoxicity and cirrhosis of liver.
4. It also precipitates "delayed chloroform poisoning" and "postanaesthetic toxemia".
5. It also produces cardiac arrest and arrhythmia.

3. Halothane (Fluothane)

- Halothane is a colourless, odourless, heavy fluid.
- It is a stable, volatile, non-inflammable and non-explosive liquid.
- 2–4% concentration is sufficient to induce anaesthesia.
- It is supplied in amber coloured bottles.

Pharmacological Actions

- A concentration of 3% is frequently used for quick induction of anaesthesia.
- All anaesthetic concentration depresses the respiration.
- Halothane inhibits salivation, laryngospasm and coughing as well.
- Halothane produces bronchodilation hence is an anaesthetic of choice in patients with the history of bronchial asthma.

Adverse Effects

- Several cardiac abnormalities.
- Hepatic damage (liver damage).

Therapeutic uses

It is used for induction and maintenance of anaesthesia.

Contraindication

- Family history of malignant hyperthermia and porphyria.

Dosage

- For adults : 2–4% concentration of halothane.
- For children : 1.5–2% concentration of halothane.

Brand name: Fluothane.

Advantages

- Induction of anaesthesia is very smooth as it has a sweet fruity odour.
- Recovery is also fast, smooth with low incidences of nausea and vomiting.
- It does not cause irritation of respiratory passage.
- It inhibits salivary secretions.
- It does not produce bronchospasm and laryngospasm hence useful in patients with bronchial asthma.

Disadvantages

- Muscular relaxation is inadequate.
- It causes respiratory, cardiovascular depression.
- Mental recovery is delayed.
- Shivering during recovery is very common.
- It is a poor analgesic.
- It is expensive, needs special apparatus for administration.

4. Nitrous Oxide (Laughing Gas)

- Nitrous oxide is a colourless gas with a slightly sweet odour.
- The gas is non-explosive and non-inflammable.
- Nitrous oxide is marketed in liquid form under 50 atmospheric pressure in royal blue steel cylinders.

Pharmacological Actions

- A mixture of nitrous oxide gas with oxygen containing 80% of it, causes unconsciousness and analgesia.
- For achieving full surgical anaesthesia with the gas, a higher concentration (up to 80%) is necessary which will cause anoxia with cerebral damage, if the inhalation continues for more than 2–3 minutes.

Adverse Effects

- Hypoxia
- Cardiac irregularities.

Therapeutic uses

1. As general anaesthetic
2. It is also employed for extraction of tooth, obstetrical analgesia and for certain painful procedures.

Dosage

For analgesia, 50% nitrous oxide mixed with 50% oxygen.

Advantages

- It is non-inflammable and non-irritant.
- It produces rapid induction and recovery.
- It has a good analgesic effect and hence can be used in dental practice.
- It is a safest anaesthetic agent.
- Incidences of nausea and vomiting are rare.

Disadvantages

- Preanaesthetic medication is required.
- Excitement may be violent.
- Special apparatus is required for administration.

5. Cyclopropane

- Cyclopropane is a very heavy colourless gas with a characteristic ether-like odour.
- Cyclopropane is marketed as a liquid, under pressure in orange coloured cylinders.
- Cyclopropane is an inflammable and explosive liquid.

Pharmacological Actions

- The quick induction of cyclopropane anaesthesia allows for a smooth and simple anaesthesia.
- Cyclopropane is a highly effective anaesthetic.
- The anaesthetic dose is sufficient to provide adequate muscular relaxation.
- The process of recovery from anaesthesia is quick.

Adverse Effects

- Cardiac abnormalities
- Cardiac arrhythmia
- Delirium
- Post-anaesthetic hypotension
- Headache.

Therapeutic uses

1. Cyclopropane is a highly effective anaesthetic.
2. It is a drug of choice for anaesthesia in cases of thoracic and abdominal operation.

Dosage

Cyclopropane IP : 30–35% concentration

Q 4. Write a note on 'intravenous anaesthetics'/'non-volatile anaesthetics'.

Intravenous/Non-volatile Anaesthetics

These are given by intravenous route for quick induction of anaesthesia for specific duration, e.g. thiopental sodium, methohexital, propandid, ketamine, althesin, etomidate.

Advantages

- Easy to administer.
- Indication is rapid and smooth.
- Post-anaesthetic complications are rare.
- Recovery is very fast.
- Respiratory and myocardial functions remain unaffected.
- No irritation of respiratory passage.

Disadvantages

- Usual stages of anaesthesia are not clear.
- Coughing, apnea is common during induction.
- Muscular relaxation is poor.
- Injection around nerve may produce palsy.

Thiopentone

- Thiopentone is a barbiturate with very high lipid solubility.
- Thiopentone sodium is a sodium salt of pentobarbitone which can be used as anaesthetic agent.

Pharmacological Actions

- Thiopentone sodium is given intravenously, usually to induce anaesthesia.
- Thiopentone is administered as 2.5–5% solution.
- When given intravenously, it is rapidly distributed and acts quickly on the brain and the effect of an initial dose of 25 mg lasts for about 15 minutes.
- Hence, it is an ultra short-acting. It is a poor analgesic.

Adverse Effects

- Respiratory depression
- Laryngospasm and bronchospasm.
- Coughing

Therapeutic uses

1. Intravenously used for induction of anaesthesia.
2. Used as a basal anaesthetic.
3. As anticonvulsant
4. As an anaesthetic in patients with history of malignant hyperthermia.

Contraindications

- Cardiovascular disease
- Dysponea
- Porphyria.

Dosage

Thiopental sodium 0.5–1 gm powder. It is used as a freshly prepared, 2.5% solution for intravenous anaesthesia, as basal anaesthesia.

Preparations and Doses of Intravenous Anaesthetics

1. Thiopentone sodium	2.5% solution	(Intraval)
2. Methohexitone	1% solution	(Brevital)
3. Propandid	4 mg/kg	
4. Ketamine	1.2 mg/kg	(Ketalar)

Q 5. Give the properties of an ideal anaesthetic agent. OR Give the requirements/ideal characteristics of an ideal general anaesthetic agent.

An ideal general anaesthetic agent should possess following properties:

a. For Patient

i. Anaesthetic agent should be pleasant to inhale without any irritation.
ii. The induction of anaesthesia should be pleasant and fast.
iii. The recovery of anaesthesia should be smooth and rapid.
iv. It should not produce any toxicity.
v. It should be non-irritant.

b. For Surgeon

i. The anaesthetic agent should produce good analgesia and adequate muscular relaxation.
ii. The capillary bleeding should be negligible.
iii. It should be nonexplosive and non-inflammable.

c. For Anaesthetist

i. It should be stable at room temperature.
ii. It should be easily controllable with a wide margin of safety.
iii. It should not cause respiratory or circulatory collapse or depression.
iv. It should be easily eliminated from the body.
v. It should not attack the materials used for anaesthesia such as rubber tubing or metal.

d. For Manufacturer

i. The cost of anaesthetic agent should be cheap.
ii. It should have no storage problem.

Q 6. What is preanaesthetic medication? Name the drugs commonly used for preanaesthetic medication.

The use of drugs before administration of anaesthetic agent to make anaesthesia safer and more aggreable to the patient is called preanaesthetic medication.

Reasons for Preanaesthetic Medication

1. To reduce anxiety, tension and nervousness.
2. To obtain synergistic effect.
3. To reduce preoperative and postoperative pains.
4. To suppress salivary and respiratory secretions.
5. To counteract adverse effects of anaesthetic agent.

Drugs Commonly used for Preanaesthetic Medication

1. **Narcotic analgesics:** These are given due to their sedative and analgesic properties, e.g. morphine 15 mg by IM.
2. **Barbiturates:** Drugs like pentobarbitone and secobarbitone are used to provide sedation and to relieve apprehension.
3. **Tranquillizers:** These agents produce calming effect and are safe muscle relaxants. They have less respiratory depression, e.g. diazepam 5–10 mg orally.
4. **Anticholinergics:** Anticholinergics such as atropine are used to reduce excessive salivary and respiratory secretions.
5. **Antiemetics:** These are used to prevent preoperative and postoperative vomiting, e.g. metoclopramide.

Q 7. What do you mean by 'basal anaesthesia'/'basal anaesthetics'? Mention the drugs used to produce based anaesthesia.

- **Basal anaesthesia:** A state of anaesthesia short of surgical anaesthesia is called basal anaesthesia.
- **Basal anaesthetics:** The drugs which are used to produce basal anaesthesia are called basal anaesthetics.
- **Uses of basal anaesthesia:** In case of extremely nervous patients and in case of hyperthyroid patients, it is always better to bring the patient in operation theatre in a state of 'basal anaesthesia'.
- The drugs used to produce basal anaesthesia are:
  1. **Thiopentone sodium:** The 2% salt is generally administered intravenously until the patient becomes unconscious.
  2. **Tribromoethanol:** It is administered as a retention enemia.
  3. **Paraldehyde:** It is also administered as a retention enemia.

Q 8. Differentiate between ether and chloroform.

Ether	*Chloroform*
1. It is a safe anaesthetic agent	1. It is not a safe anaesthetic agent
2. 10–15% concentration of ether is sufficient to produce anaesthesia.	2. 1% concentration is sufficient
3. Ether can be used during delivery to reduce labour pains	3. It is not used during labour pains due to its high toxicity
4. Ether is colourless volatile liquid, with pungent odour	4. Chloroform is a clear volatile liquid having sweet smell
5. Ether, when exposed to air, forms ether peroxides or presence of flame and forms acetic aldehydes	5. Chloroform decomposes in the phosgene gas which is toxic

Q 9. Differentiate between general anaesthetics and local anaesthetics.

General anaesthetics	*Local anaesthetics*
1. General anaesthetics are the agents which bring about loss of all modalities of sensation, particularly pain, along with a reversible loss of consciousness	1. It may be defined as any substance applied topically or by localized injection or infiltration to dull or block pain sensation
2. General anaesthesia is induced either by inhalation of valatile and gaseous anaesthetics like diethyl ether, halothane or parenteral administration of intravenous anaesthetics like thiopentone	2. Local anaesthesia is induced by topical application of drug to skin or mucous membrane or by injection into area subjected to surgical operation or injection into dural membrane of spinal cord
3. General anaesthesia is carried out before carrying out surgical operation or in obstetrics	3. Local anaesthesia is produced in short surgical operations and in dentistry
4. Care of vital organs is essential	4. Care of vital organs is not essential
5. In this case consciousness is lost	5. In this case effect is a limited area of the body
6. In this case site of action is on CNS	6. In this case site of action is on peripheral nerves
7. Examples: Ether, halothane, cyclopropane	7. Examples: Lignocaine, procaine, orthocaine

QUESTIONS: GIVE THE REASONS

Q 1. Why is chloroform not safe/good general anaesthetic agent? OR Why is chloroform not used as general anaesthetic in clinical practice?

Because:

i. Chloroform may produce toxic effects on heart, liver and kidney.
ii. It produces hepatotoxicity, cardiotoxicity, cirrhosis of liver.
iii. It also precipitates 'delayed chloroform poisoning' and 'postanaesthetic toxemia'.
iv. It also produces hypotension, cardiac arrest and arrhythmia.

Hence, because of its less margin of safety, it is not used in clinical practice.

Q 2. Why is ether a safe anaesthetic agent?

Because:

i. Ether produces smooth effects during induction of anaesthesia.
ii. Ether has sweet, fruity odour.
iii. Recovery of anaesthesia is fast, smooth.
iv. Possibility of nausea, vomiting is less.
v. It does not produce bronchospasm and laryngospasm.
vi. It is also used to reduce labour pains.

Hence, ether is a safe anaesthetic.

Q 3. Why are halothane and cyclopropane costly anaesthetics?

Because:

i. Halothane and cyclopropane are poor analgesics and poor muscle relaxants. Hence, require preanaesthetic medication which adds to the cost of therapy.
ii. Administration of halothane and cyclopropane needs special apparatus.

Hence, halothane and cyclopropane are costly anaesthetics, i.e. expensive.

Q 4. Why is ether stored in amber coloured bottles?

Because:

i. Ether is a colourless volatile liquid with pungent odour.
ii. Ether when exposed to air or moisture or light, may form ether peroxides which are very irritant.
iii. To avoid this ether is marketed in amber coloured bottles covered with black paper.

Q 5. Why is atropine (anticholinergic) used in preanaesthetic medication?

Because:

i. Some volatile anaesthetics may cause nasal irritation and increase nasal and salivary secretions which interfere with anaesthesia.
ii. Atropine is antisecretory agent thus it blocks all secretions which interefere with anaesthesia.

Q 6. Why is atropine used with ether when ether is used as a general anaesthetic?/Combination of atropine and ether is used for general anaesthesia. Why?

Because:

i. Ether vapours are irritant, which irritate respiratory, lacrimal, salivary secretions.

ii. These secretions interefere with normal respiration as well as with anaesthetic process.
iii. Atropine is an antisecretory agent, it blocks all secretions and increases anaesthetic process.

Q 7. Why is nitrous oxide called 'laughing gas'?

Because nitrous oxide when administered along with air, produces a stage of excitement, delirium and also produces amnesia. It shows laughing expressions. Hence, called laughing gas.

Q 8. Why prolonged surgery cannot be undertaken with nitrous oxide alone?

The two main disadvantages which limit the use of nitrous oxide as anaesthetic agent are:
i. Low anaesthetic potency
ii. It produces hypoxia

At the maximum safe concentration of 85%, it cannot achieve surgical stage of anaesthesia. But since it possess many good properties such as non-explosive, non-irritant, pleasant smell, marked analgesia and rapid induction, which make it a valuable basal anaesthetic to be supplemented by other more potent agents.

Objective Questions with Answers in Bold Letters

1. **Crawford Long (1842) and Morton (1846)** achieved the first satisfactory result for a general anaesthetic.
2. Cyclopropane is a **gaseous** anaesthetic.
3. Postanaesthetic toxemia is an adverse effect of **chloroform.**
4. **Nitrous oxide** is known as laughing gas.
5. Cyclopropane is stored in **orange coloured cylinders** under pressure.
6. Thiopentone sodium is used to produce **basal anaesthesia.**
7. Etomidate, althesin, ketamine, propofol are **intravenous anaesthetics.**
8. **Thiopentone** is a barbiturate with very high lipid solubility.
9. The drugs used prior to anaesthetic agent are called **preanaesthetic medications.**
10. General anaesthetics are administered by **inhalation or intravenous routes.**
11. Halothane, nitrous oxide, enflurane, ether are **inhalation anaesthetics.**
12. A state of anaesthesia short of surgical anaesthesia is called **basal anaesthesia.**
13. Paraldehyde is administered as **retention enemia.**
14. Hepatotoxicity and cardiotoxicity are the major adverse effects of **chloroform.**
15. Ether is stored in **amber coloured** bottles.
16. **Anticholinergic (atropine)** is used in preanaesthetic medication.
17. **Atropine** is antisecretory agent.

B. HYPNOTICS AND SEDATIVES

Q 1. Define and classify hypnotics and sedatives giving suitable examples.

- **Hypnotics:** The drugs which induce a sleep resembling a natural sleep are called hypnotics.
- **Sedatives:** The drugs which produce calming effects without inducing sleep or the drugs which reduce excitement are called sedatives.
- **Insomnia:** Insomnia means lack of sleep or inability to sleep.

Classification of Hypnotics and Sedatives

1. Barbiturates

These are classified as follows:

a. **Long-acting barbiturates:** Duration of action is eight hours or more, e.g. barbitone, phenobarbitone.
b. **Intermediate-acting barbiturates:** Duration of action is four hours, e.g. amylbarbitone, cyclobarbitone.
c. **Short-acting barbiturates:** Duration of action is less than four hours, e.g. hexobarbitone, secobarbitone.
d. **Ultra short-acting barbiturates:** Duration of action is less than one hour, e.g. thiopentone, methohexitone.

2. Non-barbiturates

These include:

a. **Benzodiazepines**, e.g. diazepam, nitrazepam, oxazepam.
b. **Alcohol**, e.g. chloral hydrate, ethanol.
c. **Aldehyde**, e.g. paraldehyde.
d. **Acetylated carbinols**, e.g. ethionamate.
e. **Inorganic ions**, e.g. bromides.
f. **Miscellaneous**, e.g. meprobamate, antihistaminics with sedative action, hyoscine.

Q 2. Write a note on 'barbiturates'. OR Give pharmacological actions, adverse effects, therapeutic uses, brand names of barbiturates/ phenobarbitone.

Barbiturates

Barbiturates are the derivatives of barbituric acid. The hypnotic activity of barbituric acid is due to replacement of hydrogen atoms attached to carbon atom at position 5 by alkyl or aryl radical.

Barbiturates are classified according to duration of action:

a. Long-acting barbiturates (action is for 8 hours or more), e.g. phenobarbitone.

b. Intermediate-acting barbiturates (action is for 4–8 hours), e.g. amylbarbitone, butobarbitone, pentobarbitone.
c. Short-acting barbiturates (action is less than 4 hours), e.g. secobarbitone, hexobarbitone.
d. Ultra short-acting barbiturates (IV), e.g. thiopentone sodium, methohexitone, kemithal.

Mechanism of Action

- Barbiturates also facilitate the actions of GABA at multiple sites in the CNS.
- Barbiturates increase the duration of the GABA-grated chloride channel openings.
- At high concentrations, the barbiturates may also be GABA mimetic, directly activating chloride channels.

Pharmacological Actions

I. Effect on CNS

Barbiturates produce depression of CNS.

i. **Sedation and hypnosis:** The long-acting and intermediate-acting barbiturates are used for sedation and hypnosis.
ii. **Anaesthetic effect:** Ultra short-acting barbiturates, when administered intravenously, produce basal or general anaesthesia. For example, thiopentone.
iii. **Anticonvulsant effect:** Phenobarbitone is a selective anticonvulsant drug and is used for prevention of grand mal epilepsy.
iv. **Analgesic effect:** Barbiturates increase the analgesic effect of salicylates and p-aminophenol derivatives.
v. **Respiration:** Higher doses of barbiturates depress the respiratory centre in medulla oblongata and may lead to respiratory collapse.

II. Effect on CVS

Therapeutic doses of barbiturates may cause a slight fall in BP and decrease the heart rate.

Toxic doses of barbiturates produce sustained hypotension.

III. Effect on GIT

Larger doses of barbiturates retard the peristalsis.

IV. Effect on Kidney

Barbiturates cause decrease in glomerular filtration and hence urine output decreases.

Adverse Effects

1. Intolerance—includes excitement, vomiting, headache, diarrhoea.

2. Megaloblastic anaemia
3. If administered to pregnant women, may depress the foetal respiration.
4. Tolerance
5. Drug dependence
6. Hangover
7. Habituation.

Indications/Therapeutic uses

1. Used as hypnotics to relieve insomnia
2. Used as an anticonvulsant
3. Used as a preanaesthetic medication
4. Used as a general anaesthetics, e.g. thiopentone
5. The psychiatric uses, e.g. pentobarbitone, thiopentone
6. Cause sedation in case of anxiety.

Preparations and Doses

Phenobarbitone tablet IP

Sedative dose: 15–30 mg daily

Hypnotic dose: 100–200 mg daily

Trade Names

Gardenal, Luminal, Garoin.

Contraindications

- Liver disease
- Dyspnoea
- Impaired renal function
- Respiratory distress.

Q 3. Give the signs and symptoms and treatments of 'acute barbiturate poisoning'. OR Write a note on 'acute barbiturate poisoning'.

Acute Barbiturate Poisoning

Acute barbiturate poisoning is caused due to ingestion of an overdose either accidently or with suicidal intention.

Signs and Symptoms

The patient of barbiturate poisoning shows:

i. Weak and rapid pulse
ii. Cold clammy skin
iii. Slow or rapid shallow breathing
iv. Constriction of pupils
v. Paralytic dilation develops initially
vi. Respiratory depression
vii. Peripheral vascular collapse
viii. Urinary retention.

Treatments

1. Gastric lavage
2. Endotracheal intubation
3. Alkalinization of urine
4. IV administration of fluids
5. Use of prophylactic antibiotics
6. Dialysis
7. Forced diuresis

1. Gastric Lavage

If the patient is conscious then gastric lavage is carried out by using syrup of ipecac or salt solution.

If the patient is unconscious then gastric aspiration is carried out by inserting tube into the stomach.

2. Endotracheal Intubation

It is performed when respiration is inadequate and also to remove secretions from respiratory tract.

Adequate ventilation is of great importance in barbiturate poisoning.

3. Forced Diuresis

In this step, diuretics such as frusemide and mannitol are used in barbiturate poisoning to increase the flow and excretion of urine. This may lead to increase in excretion of barbiturates. Forced diuresis is most useful in poisoning due to phenobarbitone, barbitone, etc.

4. Alkalinization of Urine

Alkalinization of urine prevents tubular reabsorption of barbiturates by ionization of filtered barbiturates. This increases the excretion of barbiturates.

Sodium bicarbonate is used for alkalinization of urine.

5. Intravenous Administration of Fluid

Intravenous fluids are given in sufficient quantity to prevent dehydration. They are also useful for the maintenance of blood volume.

6. Use of Prophylactic Antibiotics

The antibiotics are used only when there is a possibility of infection due to catheterization of urinary bladder, etc.

7. Dialysis

Elimination of barbiturate from the body can be increased by peritoneal dialysis and haemodialysis.

Q 4. Write a note on 'benzodiazepines as a hypnotic and sedative'.

Benzodiazepines

- It is a group of structurally related drugs which acts on the CNS.
- The main site of action is limbic system, the region and brain concerned with emotions and anxiety.

- The drugs belong to benzodiazepine are effective for treatment of anxiety, anticonvulsant and central muscle relaxants.
- Benzodiazepines are inactivated by liver and excreted in the liver.
- Based on their duration of action, benzodiazepines are divided as:
  - i. Short acting, e.g. triazolam, flurazepam.
  - ii. Medium acting, e.g. alprazepam, lorazepam.
  - iii. Long acting, e.g. diazepam, chlordizepoxide, clonazepam, nitrazepam.

Mechanism of Action

- GABA (gamma-aminobutyric acid) is the major inhibitory neurotransmitter in CNS.
- Benzodiazepines increase the efficiency of GABA ergic synaptic inhibition.
- The effect of benzodiazepines is to enhance the response to GABA, by facilitating the opening of GABA activated chloride channel.

Pharmacological Actions

1. Reduction of anxiety and aggression.
2. Depression of cognitive and psychomotor function.
3. **Sedation and induction of sleep:** At higher dose, benzodiazepines change sleep pattern.
   - Induction of normal sleep (latency of sleep is reduced).
   - The duration of stage 2 NREM sleep is increased.
   - The duration of slow-wave sleep is decreased.
4. **Skeletal muscle relaxant effect**, e.g. diazepam relaxes muscle spasticity by presynaptic inhibition in the spinal cord.
5. **Anticonvulsant effect:** Especially diazepam, lorazepam, clonazepam, nitrazepam.
6. **Respiratory system and CVS:** Minimal depressant effects in therapeutic doses.

Therapeutic uses/Clinical uses/Indications

1. As hypnotics and sedatives
2. As anticonvulsants
3. As preanaesthetic medication
4. As antianxiety agents
5. As good muscle relaxants
6. As tranquillizers
7. To treat insomnia
8. In acute alcohol withdrawl
9. In chronic muscle spasm and spasticity.

Adverse Effects

i. **Tolerance:** Physical and psychological dependance.

ii. **Withdrawal symptoms:** Anxiety, rebound insomnia, anorexia, tremors and convulsion.
iii. Hangover, drowsiness, sleep tendency, confusion especially in long acting drugs.
iv. Light headedness, ataxia, vertigo, blurred vision.

Contraindications

- Respiratory depression
- Acute pulmonary insufficiency, sleep apnoea.
- Severe hepatic impairment
- Myasthenia gravis.

Dosage

1. Diazepam : 5–40 mg daily (valium, calmpose)
2. Nitrazepam : 5–10 mg daily (hypnotex)
3. Lorazepam : 5–10 mg daily (ativan)
4. Chlordiazepoxide : 5–10 mg daily (librium)

QUESTION: GIVE THE REASONS

Q 1. Why is sodium bicarbonate given in barbiturate poisoning?

i. Sodium bicarbonate is an alkaline, and barbiturates are the derivatives of barbituric acid.
ii. In barbiturate poisoning, unionized barbiturate is reabsorbed into the body and increases toxicity.
iii. Sodium bicarbonate increases alkalinisation of urine and there is an ionisation of barbiturates.
iv. Ionised barbiturates are not reabsorbed by tubules and increases its excretion.
v. Sodium bicarbonate increases the excretion of barbiturates and hence, it is used in barbiturate poisoning.

Objective Questions with Answers in Bold Letters

1. The condition of lack of sleep is called **insomnia**.
2. **Hypnotics** are the agents that induces sleep resembling natural sleep.
3. **Sedatives** are the drugs which reduces excitement.
4. Thiopentone and methohexione are **ultra short-acting barbiturates**.
5. **Sodium bicarbonate** is used as antidote in acute barbiturate poisoning.
6. **GABA** is the major inhibitory neurotransmitter in CNS.
7. **Barbiturates** are the derivatives of barbituric acid.

8. Calmpose is a brand name of **diazepam**.
9. REM sleep means **rapid eye movement sleep**.
10. NREM sleep means **non-rapid eye movement sleep**.
11. Automatism is a stage which occurs in case of **barbiturates**.
12. Daily dose of diazepam is **5–40 mg**.

C. ANTICONVULSANT DRUGS (ANTIEPILEPTIC DRUGS)

Q 1. What is epilepsy? Explain various types of epilepsy.

Epilepsy/Seizures

It is a chronic convulsive disorder characterised by sudden disturbance of consciousness usually but not always with characteristic body movements and sometimes with autonomic hyperactivity.

- The term epilepsy is derived from the Greek word *epilabanein* which means to seize (i.e. to take sudden possession).
- Epilepsy is the most common neurological disorders characterized by paroxysmal cerebral dysrhythmia.
- Seizures are symptoms of disturbed electrical activity in the brain characterized by episodes of abnormal, excessive and synchronus discharge of a group of neurons within the brain that causes involuntary movement, sensation or thought.

Types of Epilepsy

1. **Grand mal epilepsy:** It involves a sudden loss of consciousness and major convulsions consisting of spasms of the whole body followed by jerky movements. Convulsions are followed by generalised CNS depression.
2. **Temporal lobe epilepsy:** It consists of sudden attacks of altered behaviour and emotions. Convulsions are absent. The entire attack consists of abnormalities of behaviour.
3. **Focal cortical epilepsy:** It consists of convulsions of single limb or a group of muscles.
4. **Minor epilepsy:** It consists of loss of consciousness without convulsions.
5. **Petit mal epilepsy:** It consists of impairment of consciousness associated with eyelid blinking (insensitivity of light).
6. **Myoclonic epilepsy:** It consists of isolated clonic jerks.
7. **Infantile epilepsy:** It occurs in infants and consists of mental deterioration.
8. **Motor epilepsy:** It involves involuntary movements of thumb, angles of mouth, movements of half side of the body may be affected like paralysis.
9. **Hypsarrhythmia:** It occurs in infants and consists of falling spell, head dropping and myoclonic jerks.

Q 2. Define and classify anticonvulsants/antiepileptic drugs.

Anticonvulsants

The drugs which are used in the treatment of convulsions/epilepsy are called anticonvulsants/antiepileptics.

Classification

1. **Drugs used in grand mal epilepsy**, e.g. phenytoin, methoin, phenobarbitone, primidone, carbamazepine.
2. **Drugs used in petit mal epilepsy**, e.g. tridione, paradione, phensuximide, ethosuximide.
3. **Drugs effective in psychomotor epilepsy**, e.g. phenytoin, primidone, tridione.
4. **Focal coritcal or jacksonian epilepsy**, e.g. phenytoin, methoin, phenobarbitone, primidone.
5. **Status epilepticus**, e.g. diazepam, paraldehyde, thiopentone.

Q 3. Describe 'phenytoin' as an anticonvulsant drug.

Phenytoin (Diphenyl Hydantoin)

It is a primary drug in the treatment of epilepsy.

Mechanism of Action (Antiepileptic Activity)

- Phenytoin exerts a selective antiepileptic action. This drug generally inhibits the spread of convulsions in the brain and shortens the duration after its discharge.
- The phenytoin decreases the neuronal sodium concentration which leads to reduction in the post-tetanic potentiation (PTP) and increase in the neuronal potassium concentration.
- The reduction in PTP by phenytoin stops the spread of convulsive discharge in the brain.

Adverse Reactions

1. Intolerance, skin rash, jaundice
2. Headache, confusion, hallucination
3. GIT irritation, nausea, vomiting
4. Megaloblastic anaemia
5. Cardiovascular collapse
6. Severe CNS depression
7. Ataxia, vertigo, liver damage.

Therapeutic uses

1. In treatment of grand mal epilepsy
2. In treatment of temporal lobe epilepsy
3. In focal cortical epilepsy
4. In cardiac arrhythmia
5. In trigeminal neuralgia.

Contraindications

- Porphyria
- Sinoatrial block
- Stokes-Adams syndrome

Preparation

Phenytoin tablet IP

Dose: 50–100 mg twice daily

Trade Names

Eptoin, Epileptin.

Q 4. Write the properties of an ideal antiepileptic agent.

1. It should be effective in all varieties of epilepsy.
2. It should have quick action and long duration of action.
3. It should have minimum side effects and non-addicting.
4. It should be orally effective.
5. It must be cheap and easily available.

Q 5. What is status epilepticus? Give its treatments.

Status epilepticus is a condition in which the epileptic attacks follow each other continuously.

The term *status epilepticus* is used to indicate repeated grand mal epileptic attacks without recovery of consciousness between the attacks.

The status epilepticus is a medical emergency and such patient must be hospitalized for proper treatment.

Treatments

1. Glucose saline is given intravenously.
2. Respiration is supported.
3. Diazepam is given intravenously for controlling convulsions.
4. Hypotension and respiratory depression may be watched carefully.
5. Paraldehyde is also given as an alternative in the dose of 5–10 ml by IM.

Q 6. Give the major use, brand name, dose of the following anticonvulsants.

Drug	*Brand name*	*Uses*	*Dose*	*Route*
1. Phenytoin	Dilantin	Grand mal epilepsy, status epilepticus	300–400 mg daily in divided doses	Oral
2. Primidone	Mysoline	Grand mal epilepsy, psychomotor epilepsy	125 mg daily for 3 days, 250 mg q.i.d.	Oral
3. Trimethadione	Tridione, Troxidone	Petit mal epilepsy	300 mg t.i.d. maintenance 2–3 gm/day	Oral
4. Paramethadione	Paradione	Petit mal epilepsy	300–600 mg t.i.d.	Oral
5. Ethosuximide	Zarontin	Petit mal epilepsy	500 mg/day initially, increased up to 1500 mg/day	Oral

Contd...

Contd...

Drug	*Brand name*	*Uses*	*Dose*	*Route*
6. Methosuximide	Celontin	Petit mal, psychomotor epilepsy	Initially 300 mg/day for a week, increased to 1000 mg/day	Oral
7. Carbamozepine	Tegretol, Mazetol	Trigeminal neuralgia, psychomotor epilepsy	100–200 mg twice daily, maintenance 400–800 mg/day	Oral
8. Sodium valproate	Epilim	Grand mal, petit mal epilepsy	1200–1500 mg/day in divided doses	Oral
9. Phenobarbitone	Gardenal, Luminal, Dilantin-P	Grand mal epilepsy	30–20 mg/day in divided doses	Oral

QUESTIONS: GIVE THE REASONS

Q 1. While treating the patient of epilepsy, the dose of drug should be reduced slowly? OR During the treatment of epilepsy, drug should be discontinued or withdrawn gradually, why? OR Why antiepileptics should not be withdrawn abruptly?

Because:

i. If antiepileptic drugs are discontinued suddenly, individual may suffer from rebound epileptic attack, which may be severe than previous one.

ii. The antiepileptic drugs show withdrawal symptoms such as delusions and hallucinations.

iii. All antiepileptic drugs are quite sedative in nature.

Hence, to reduce above side effects, the dose of drug is reduced slowly.

Q 2. Why is phenobarbitone used in epilepsy?

Because phenobarbitone inhibits the spread of convulsive discharge in the brain and exerts an antiepileptic effect. Due to this property it is used in epilepsy.

Q 3. Generally combination of phenytoin and phenobarbitone is used in the treatment of grand mal epilepsy.

i. Phenytoin prevents the spread of grand mal and other epileptic seizures.

ii. Phenytoin prevents the spread of abnormal electrical activity but does not seem to abolish the focus.

iii. Phenobarbitone reduces both the formation of focus and its spread.

iv. Phenytoin causes effux of sodium from cerebral neurones and thus stabilise their cell membranes for a particular electrical charge and prevents PTP.

v. Phenobarbitone increases the post-synaptic responses to the inhibitory transmitter GABA.

vi. The combination also considerable reduces the systemic toxicity due to decrease in the proportion of individual drug. This combination has synergistic action. Hence generally, combination of phenytoin and phenobarbitone is used in the treatment of grand mal epilepsy.

Objective Questions with Answers in Bold Letters

1. Carbamazepine belongs to **iminostilbene group**.
2. Epilepsy is a **neurological** disorder.
3. **Epilepsy** is also known as seizure/convulsion.
4. **Grand mal epilepsy** is also known as major epilepsy.
5. Phenytoin is a drug of choice in **grand mal epilepsy**.
6. **Diazepam** is a drug of choice in status epilepticus.
7. Primidone is an anticonvulsant which is structurally related to **phenobarbitone**.
8. Petit mal seizures are also known as **absence seizures**.

D. ANTIANXIETY DRUGS/ANXIOLYTICS

Q 1. What do you mean by anxiety? Define and classify antianxiety drugs.

Anxiety

It is an emotional state characterized by intense, excessive persistent worry and fear about defined or undefined future threat.

Anxiety is also associated with physical changes such as insomnia, hypersomnia, anorexia and weight loss.

Symptoms

- Feeling nervous, restless
- Increased heart rate
- Sweating
- Feeling tired
- Inability to concentrate on any other thing than the present worry.

Causes

- Difficult experience in childhood, adolescence or adulthood.
- Stress
- Trauma
- Physical/emotional abuse

Antianxiety Drugs

The drugs which are used in the treatment of anxiety are called antianxiety drugs.

Classification

1. **Minor tranquillizers:** Benzodiazepines: Diazepam, chlordiazepoxide, lorazepam, oxazepam and alprazolam.
2. **Antidepressants:** Further classified into the following classes:
   a. *Monoamine oxidase (MAO) inhibitors:* Isocarboxazid, nialamide
   b. *Tricyclic compounds:* Impiramine, desipramine, amitriptyline
   c. *Selective serotonin reuptake inhibitors:* Fluoxetin, citalopram
   d. *Lithium carbonate.*

Q 2. Describe any two antianxiety agents (minor tranquillizers).

Antianxiety Drugs

1. Benzodiazepines

Pharmacological actions:

- Chlordiazepoxide is a tranquillizer which has to a great replaced with meprobamate.
- Animal studies have shown that chlordiazepoxide has sedative, anti-convulsant and skeletal muscle relaxant properties.
- Chlordiazepoxide is rapidly absorbed from the GIT and peak blood levels are reached within 2–4 hours.
- The drug is excreted slowly and its plasma half life is 20–40 hours.

Therapeutic uses

1. Symptomatic relief anxiety
2. To reduce anxiety of psychosis
3. In prophylaxis of migraine
4. To treat acute symptoms of alcohol withdrawal
5. Effective in treatment of musculoskeletal diseases.

Adverse Reactions

- Drowsiness
- Ataxia
- Lethargy
- Syncope

Dosage

1. Chlordiazepoxide tab 20–100 mg daily (librium)
2. Other benzodiazepines used an anxiety includes:
   Oxazepam (30–60 mg) : 2–3 divided doses
   Diazepam (5–30 mg)
   Lorazepam (1–6 mg)
   Alprazolam (0.25–1 mg)

2. Meprobamate

- Meprobamate is highly effective antianxiety agent and mild skeletal muscle relaxants.

- It produce mild sedation and relaxation.
- It is indicated for the relief of anxiety and tension.
- Meprobamate is an anxiolytic drug.
- Meprobamate is minor tranquillizer but has largely been replaced by benzodiazepine.
- Meprobamate is of little value in the treatment of psychoses.
- Tolerance may develop rapidly and a physical dependance may develop for the drug if it is taken for prolonged periods.
- Withdrawal symptoms appear in 95% of the patients when the drug is discontinued.
- Convulsions, delirium and grand mal seizures may be precipitated on withdrawal of a drug.

Adverse Effects

- Drowsiness
- Slurred speech
- Tolerance
- Ataxia
- Blood dyscrasias
- Depression
- Allergic reactions
- Euphoria
- Psychological dependance.

Indications/Therapeutic uses

1. Used in anxiety and neurosis.
2. As a hypnotic and sedative.
3. Used during withdrawal of alcohol.

Dosage

Meprobamate tablet :1200–1600 mg daily in divided doses

Brand Name: Miltown.

E. ANTIDEPRESSANTS/PSYCHOANALEPTICS

Q 1. What do you mean by 'depression'? Define and classify antidepressant drugs.

Depression

- Depression is a mental illness characterized by pathological changes in mood.
- Depression is a sadness, though possibly intense, it is usually of short duration.

Causes

Decrease the level of excitatory neurotransmitters (adrenaline, noradrenaline and serotonin).

Symptoms

1. Loss of pleasure in usual activities (anhedonia).
2. Sleep disturbances

3. Persistently sad, anxious, or empty moods
4. Feelings of helplessness, guilt, or worthlessness
5. Fatigue or decreased energy
6. Loss of memory, concentration, or decision-making capability
7. Restlessness, irritability
8. Change in appetite or weight

Antidepressant drugs: These are the agents that used to treat the depression.

Classification of Antidepressants/Psychoanaleptics/Mood Elevators/ Thymoleptics

1. **Tricyclic antidepressants**, e.g. imipramine, desipramine, amitriptyline, nortriptyline, doxepin.
2. **Monoamine oxidase inhibitors (MAOIs)**, e.g. isocarboxazid, nialamide, phenelzine, pargyline, tranylcypromine.
3. **Mood stabilizers**, e.g. lithium carbonate, mainserin.

Q 2. Write a note on •'MAO inhibitors'.

MAO inhibitors mean monoamine oxidase inhibitors. The drugs which inhibit the actions of monoamine oxidase enzyme are known as monoamine oxidase inhibitors. For example, phenelzine, pargyline, isocarboxazid, tranylcypromine.

- MAO inhibitors are a heterogenous group of drugs which block oxidation of naturally occurring amines.
- MAO inhibitors have a limited role in the management of depression.

Mechanism of Action

The enzyme monoamine oxidase is present intracellularly in most of the tissues. The highest concentration is found in liver, within the brain and its important function is to oxidise active biogenic amines, 5-HT, noradrenaline and dopamine.

These amines are normally stored in granules in neurons and are liberated by nerve stimuli.

MAO inhibitors inhibit the action of MAO enzymes which may lead to accumulation of these monoamines in the brain. MAO inhibitors prevent oxidation of catecholamine and histamine and increase functional availability of these monoamines in the brain. MAO inhibitors are effective in the treatment of mental depression of man because these drugs produce their pharmacological action by increasing the level of active amines like 5-HT.

Adverse Effects

1. Headache, excitement
2. Disturbed sleep
3. Hyperthermia
4. Convulsions
5. Sudden increase in BP
6. Constipation
7. Severe jaundice.

Therapeutic uses

1. As antidepressants
2. As antihypertensive agents
3. They potentiate the action of barbiturates, morphine and anaesthetics.

Preparation and Doses

1. Phenelzine sulphate tablet

   Dose: 50–60 mg daily orally **Trade name:** Nardil
2. Isocarboxazid tablet

   Dose: 10–30 mg daily orally **Trade name:** Morphan
3. Tranylcypromine tablet

   Dose: 10–30 mg daily **Trade name:** Parnate.

Q 3. Write a note on 'tricyclic antidepressants/imipramine.

Tricyclic Antidepressants

- These compounds inhibit the reuptake of norepinephrine and serotonin into adrenergic neurons.
- These compounds may be subdivided into:
  a. Tertiary amines: Amitriptyline, doxepin, imipramine, trimipramine.
  b. Secondary amines: Desipramine, amoxapine, protriptyline.
- All tricyclic compounds display anticholinergic activity.
- These compounds are more specifically effective in treating patients with endogenous depression.
- In combination therapy with phenothiazines or lithium carbonate may be beneficial in treating depression of schizophrenia or severe anxiety.

Impramine: Impramine is a dibenzazepine derivative and is commonly used as tricyclic antidepressant drug.

Pharmacological Actions

- **Behavioural effects:** It has antidepressant properties comparable to MAO inhibitors, but its mechanism of action is distinct. It also has some anxiolytic properties.
- **Central nervous system:** Drowsiness and lightheadedness are caused by a single dose. It also has sedative properties and improves sleep. It reduces the seizure threshold; thus, it should be used with caution in individuals who have seizures. Sedation and trouble concentrating and thinking are caused by repeated doses of the medication. The medication has no effect on breathing at therapeutic levels. Drug addiction is a rare occurrence.

- **Autonomic nervous system:** It has significant anticholinergic effects, such as dry mouth, constipation, palpitation and so on.
- **Cardiovascular system:** In anaesthetized animals, it reduces blood pressure. In humans, therapeutic doses cause moderate hypotension. Cardiac arrhythmia is caused by taking too much of the medicine.
- **Adverse effects:**
- **Anticholinergic disturbances:** Dry mouth, difficulty in adapting, tachycardia, difficulty in micturition, impotence, constipation and delayed ejaculation are all side effects of these medicines. Hyperpyrexia is a rare side effect.
- **CNS:** Tiredness, lethargy, headaches and drowsiness are common side effects. Tremors, muscle jerks, ataxia and hyperreflexia are also side effects of the drug.
- **Cardiovascular system:** Tachycardia, cardiac arrhythmia and hypotension are all possible side effects. In some cases, heart failure has been documented.
- It produces allergic reactions such as skin rashes, photosensitivity, cholestatic jaundice, edema and agranulocytosis.

Therapeutic uses/Indications

- It is indicated in phobic and obsessional states.
- It is used to treat anxiety disorders.
- It is used to treat pains due to its analgesic property.
- It is used to treat hyperactivity and disturbed attention.
- It is used to treat allergic conjunctivitis.
- To treat enuresis (bed wetting in children).

Preparations

- Imipramine tablet
- Imipramine mixture
- Imipramine injection
- Imipramine capsule.

Brand names: Antidep, Depranil, Depsonil, Imrotab.

Contraindications

- Recent myocardial infarction
- Severe liver disease.
- Arrhythmias

Dosage

Phobic and obsessional states: Initially 25 mg daily at bed time by mouth and may be increased over two weeks to 100–150 mg daily.

Q 4. Explain 'lithium carbonate' as antidepressant drug.

Lithium Carbonate

- Lithium carbonate is used for prophylactic treatment of recurrent maniac and depressive episodes.

- Lithium carbonate causes depletion of intraneural sodium and stabilises the neuronal membrane.
- It also prevents the release of norepinephrine.

Adverse Effects

- Nausea
- Diarrhoea
- Blurred vision
- Anorexia
- Hypothyroidism
- Convulsions
- Stomach irritation
- Thirst
- Coma.

Therapeutic uses

1. In treatment and prophylaxis of mania.
2. In prophylaxis of bipolar disorder and recurrent depression.
3. In treatment of prophylaxis of schizophrenia.

Contraindications

- Renal impairment
- Addison's disease.

Dosage

Lithium carbonate tablet : 250–2000 mg daily in divided doses
Brand names: Lithocarb, Licab.

QUESTION: GIVE THE REASONS

Q 1. Why eating of cheese is forbidden in patients with MAO inhibitor therapy?

- Cheese, butter, chocolates, bananas contain tyramine. Tyramine is metabolised in the liver by the enzyme monoamine oxidase.
- If individual is on MAO inhibitor therapy, then MAO inhibitors inhibit the detoxification or metabolism of tyramine.
- Thus, tyramine is not metabolised and it gets accumulated in the body.
- This tyramine causes release of noradrenaline from its binding sites.
- Increased level of noradrenaline causes hypertensive crisis.
- Therefore, eating of cheese is forbidden while on MAO inhibitor therapy.

F. ANTIPSYCHOTICS

Q 1. What are different psychic disorders/psychological disorders/ mental disorders?

Types of Psychic/Mental Disorders

Psychosis: It means a mental condition characterized by disturbances in mental functions.

- It is a psychic condition, which involves marked impairment of behaviour with a serious inability to think.
- Mental diseases have always been puzzling and frightening things.

- Psychosis can be defined as the psychotic illness with serious distortion of thought, behaviour and capacity to recognize reality and of perception and patient unable to meet the ordinary demand of life.

Psychoses may be of two categories:

a. **Organic psychosis:** It involves memory disturbances, clouding of consciousness, congestive disorders, like delirium and dementia with psychotic features.
   Prominent features are confusion, disorientation, defective memory, disorganized thoughts and behaviour. They may be due to endocrinal abnormalities or head injuries.
b. **Functional psychosis:**
   i. *Maniac:* Disturbance of mood, reduced sleep, hyperactivity, uncontrollable thoughts and speech, violent behaviour.
   ii. *Schizophrenia:* It is also known as split mind condition. It involves splitting of perception and interpretation from reality and inability to think. Disturbed emotions and motor behaviour.
   iii. *Hallucination:* A sensation of false perception without sensory stimulus.
   iv. *Anxiety:* It involves feeling of fear, apprehension.
c. **Neurosis:** It is a termed used to denote less severe form of psychosis.
d. **Depression:** It is a common psychiatric disorder characterized by a feeling of misery, apathy, hopelessness, ugliness, loss of appetite, insomnia, anorexia, alternation in moods, activities, etc.

Q 2. Define the terms with examples.

a. Antipsychotics/Psychotropics/Psychoactive Drugs

The drugs which are used in the treatment of psychic disorders are called antipsychotics or psychoactive drugs. For example, chlorpromazine, reserpine, haloperidol.

b. Antianxiety Agents/Anxiolytics/Minor Tranquillizers

The drugs which are used to reduce anxiety states and nervousness are called antianxiety agents. For example, diazepam, nitrazepam, oxazepam.

c. Antidepressants (Mood Elevators)

The drugs which improve the moods of depressed individuals are called antidepressants. For example, imipramine, desipramine, amitriptyline, nortriptyline.

d. Tranquillizers

The drugs which produce calming and quietening effect on the individuals are called tranquillizers. For example, chlorpromazine, haloperidol.

Q 3. Define and classify antipsychotics/psychoactive drugs/psychotropic drugs/tranquillizers with suitable examples.

Psychotropic/Antipsychotic Drugs

The drugs which are used to treat psychiatric disorders are called psychotropic drugs.

Classification

A. **Typical antipsychotics:** These drugs act on the dopaminergic system, blocking the dopamine type 2(D_2) receptors.
   a. ***Phenothiazines***, e.g. chlorpromazine, trifluoperazine.
   b. ***Butyrophenone derivatives***, e.g. haloperidol, droperidol.
   c. ***Thiothixene derivatives***, e.g. thiothixene, chlorprothixene.
   d. ***Miscellaneous***, e.g. reserpine (Rauwolfia alkaloids).

B. **Atypical antipsychotics:** For example, clonazepine, risperidone.

Q 4. Write a note on 'major tranquillizers'/'phenothiazines'.

Major Tranquillizers/Phenothiazines

Chlorpromazine

- It is a phenothiazine derivative.
- It produces many pharmacological actions hence, it is called by the trade name 'Largactil'.

Pharmacological Actions

1. **Behavioural Effects:**
   - In patients, with major psychosis, it produces psychomotor slowing, emotional quietening, diminishing anxiety without affecting wakefullness.
   - The drug produces antipsychotic effect by blocking the receptors of dopamine and norepinephrine in the brain.
   - The antipsychotic action is due to competitive blockade of dopaminergic receptors in limbic system.
2. **Effect of ANS:** It has central depressant action on hypothalamic centre controlling sympathetic activity.
3. **Effect on CVS:** It produces hypotension because of depression of hypothalamus leading to decrease in sympathetic tone. It produces vasodilation.
4. **Antiemetic effect:** It depresses CTZ in the medulla and acts as a powerful antiemetic.
5. **Effect on temperature regulating centre:** It decreases temperature by adrenergic blocking effect which leads to vasodilation resulting in heat loss.

Adverse Effects

1. Skin rash, dermatitis
2. Parkinsonism
3. Excitement, restlessness
4. Tachycardia
5. Constipation
6. Hypotension
7. Aplastic anemia
8. Menstrual irregularities.

Therapeutic uses

1. In the treatment of schizophrenia.
2. In senile psychosis (aged).
3. In the treatment of maniac depressive psychosis.
4. For the treatment of behavioural disorders in children.
5. It acts as an antiemetic by acting on CTZ.

Preparation and Doses

Chlorpromazine tablet IP
Dose: 200–800 mg daily
Brand name: Largactil

Contraindications

- Bone marrow depression
- Pheochromocytoma.

Q 5. Explain the details of 'reserpine' as a tranquillizer.

Reserpine

It is a principal alkaloid of *Rauwolfia serpentina.*

Mechanism of Action (Tranquillizing Action)

Reserpine produces depletion of 5-HT and catecholamines (adrenaline and noradrenaline) from the brain and peripheral sites. This depletion of monoamines is necessary for its tranquillizing action.

Therapeutic uses

1. As antipsychotic (tranquillizer).
2. As an antihypertensive agent.
3. Used in the treatment of snake bite.

Preparation and Dose

Reserpine tablet IP
Dose: 0.25 mg daily
Trade name: Serpasil.

Q 6. Explain the terms and give the drugs of choice.

1. Schizophrenia

- It is a split mind condition characterized by disturbed thinking, emotional withdrawal from surrounding, delusions, and hallucination.

- The mental functions of schizophrenic patient are sufficiently impaired to interfere with his capacity to meet the ordinary demands of life.

Drug Treatment

Chlorpromazine, reserpine.

2. Motion Sickness

Motion sickness can develop during any form of travel but is mainly due to repetitive and rhythmic changes in speed or direction of travel.

It starts with a brief period of euphoria and then followed by uneasiness. The face becomes pale and a cold sweat breakout, nausea, salivation, and vomiting occurs with headache.

Drug Treatment

Scopolamine, promethazine, cyclizine, d-amphetamine.

Q 7. What is mania? Write in brief about antimanic drugs (mood stabilizers).

Mania

It is also known as bipolar disorder. It causes serious shift in mood energy thinking and behaviour—from the highs of mania on one extreme, to the lows of depression on the other.

Symptoms

1. Sleeping very little, but feeling extremely energetic.
2. Talking so rapidly that others cannot keep up.
3. Feeling unusually 'high' and optimistic or extremely irritable.
4. Highly distractible, unable to concentrate.

Antimanic drugs: These are the agents that are used to stabilize the mood of individuals is called antimanic drugs.

Lithium

Mechanism of action: Lithium decreases the body sodium content. It is equally distributed in and out of the cell and effects its ionic environment. It decreases NA and DA release in brain.

Pharmacological Actions

1. It inhibits the ADH (antidiuretic hormone) action on distal tubule and produce polyuria and thirst.
2. It has insulin-like action on glucose metabolism.

Therapeutic uses

1. Mainly used to treat manic episodes
2. Treatment of bipolar disorder.

Adverse Effects

Increased thirst and urination, polydipsia, nausea, weakness, drowsiness and fatigue.

QUESTIONS: GIVE THE REASONS

Q 1. Why is chlorpromazine 'called 'Largactil'?

Because chlorpromazine shows a large number of pharmacological actions as follows:

i. It causes sedation.
ii. In psychotic patients cause tranquillizing effect.
iii. It has an antiemetic effect.
iv. It causes hypothermia by acting on hypothalamus.
v. It promotes lactation in women and blocks ovulation.
vi. It has weak antihistaminic activity.
vii. In normal individuals, it causes emotional quietening.

Due to all these actions, chlorpromazine is called Largactil.

Q 2. Why is chlorpromazine not effective in the vomiting of motion sickness?

Because:

i. Motion sickness means vomiting induced during travelling, may be due to repetitive and rhythmic changes in the speed or direction of travel.
ii. Motion sickness is caused by stimulation of vestibular nucleus but not by CTZ.
iii. Chlorpromazine is antiemetic drug and it prevents the vomiting induced due to stimulation of CTZ only.

Thus, chlorpromazine is not effective in motion sickness.

Q 3. Why reserpine is not useful in immediate quietening of manic patients?

i. Reserpine is an antipsychotic drug.
ii. It causes depletion of serotonin and catecholamines from the brain and peripheral sites which results in tranquillizing action.
iii. Reserpine stimulates the CNS excessively leading to firing of all central neurons synchronously developing epilepsy.
iv. This is followed by severe mental depression resulting in suicidal tendencies.
v. Therefore, reserpine is not useful in immediate quietening of manic patients.

G. NOOTROPIC AGENTS

Q 1. What are nootropics? Explain various nootropic agents.

Nootropics

Nootropics are the drugs supplements and other substances that are claimed to improve cognitive function, particularly executive functions such as attention, memory, creativity or motivation, in healthy individuals.

Explanation

- Nootropics are 'smart drugs' that can boost brain performance.
- They are sometimes called cognition enhancers or memory enhancing substances.
- Nootropics are used to boost memory, improve concentration thereby focus creativity and postpone fatigue.
- The word nootropics is derived from the Greek words *nous* → means mind, *trepein* → means to bend or turn. Thus, nootropics means 'monitoring mind'.
- Nootropics can treat number of neurodegenerative and neuropsychiatric disorders.
- Nootropics are available in natural and synthetic forms:
  a. **Natural phytoconstituents:** These include caffeine, L-theanine, creatine, *Bacopa monnieri* (Brahmi), *Rhodiola rosea*, *Panax ginseng*, *Ginkgo biloba*, etc.
  b. **Synthetic agents:** These include piracetam, citicoline, levetiracetam, armodafinil, ampakines, cerebrolysin, phenibut, modafinil, selegiline, semax, inositol, etc.

A. **Natural phytoconstituents:** These include:

1. *Caffeine:* It is most widely consumed psychoactive substance in the world. It is found in coffee, tea cola nuts. It is added to many sodas, energy drinks and medications. It is taken as supplement either alone or in combination with others. Caffeine works by blocking adenosine receptors in the brain, making person feel less tired. Low to moderate caffeine intake 40–300 mg enhance alertness and attention. It reduces reaction time. It is especially useful for people with fatigue.
2. *L-Theanine:* It is a naturally occurring amino acid found in tea. Studies have shown that taking 200 mg of L-theanine has calming effect without causing drowsiness. Even 50 mg have been found to increase α-waves in the brain, linked to creativity. It is more effective when taken with caffeine (tea contains both caffeine and L-theanine).
3. *Creatine:* It is an amino acid required for protein synthesis. It is popular body building material that promotes growth. In brain, it combines with

phosphate and form a substance, useful as energy fuel for brain. It enhances short-term memory and reasoning skills especially in stressed people. Consumption of 5 g per day has been shown to be safe.

4. *Bacopa monnieri:* It is an ancient herb used in ayurvedic medicine. It improves brain, functions, speeds up information processing in the brain and reduce reaction time along with improvement in memory. The active compounds found in it are known as becosides which protect the brain from oxidative stress. 300–600 mg per day should be taken for several months to achieve maximum benefit.
5. *Rhodiola rosea:* Adaptogenic herbs that help to handle stress more effectively and improve mood, reduce feeling of burnouts in both anxious and highly stressed individuals. It relieves mental fatigue and enhance feeling of well-being in college students during stressful examination times.
6. *Panax ginseng:* Ancient medicinal plant that boosts brain function. Taking single dose of 200–400 mg of *Panax ginseng* has been shown to reduce brain fatigue.

B. **Synthetic compounds:** These include:

1. *Piracetam:* A nootropic agent which is derivative of γ-aminobutyric acid (GABA) used in Europe as enhancer of cognitive skills. Its exact mechanism is not clearly known but is supposed to act by enhancing acetylcholine and glutamate transmission. It improves memory and learning in humans.
2. *Citicoline:* A psychostimulant/nootropic agent that stimulates both motor and sensory systems. It has been observed that, the intake of citicoline has elicited changes in EEG and EMG, consistent with aurosal of consciousness. The effects are attributable to brain adrenergic, especially dopaminergic neurotransmitter systems.
3. *Levetiracetam:* A newer anticonvulsant that is claimed to improve cognition, i.e. showing nootropic effects.

Q 2. State important features of nootropics.

Important Features of Nootropics

- Nootropics are class of cognitive enhancing supplements that enhance concentration and boost memory.
- They are also referred to as 'smart drugs' as they are concerned with intelligence, motivation and mental strength.
- Long-term safety data about nootropics is not available, clinical research data suggest that only certain stimulants used in low doses can enhance cognition in general population.
- Nootropics act as direct or indirect agonists of dopamine, adrenoceptor or both in prefrontal cortex.

- Nootropics show signs of neuropreservation and neuroprotection.
- Some nootropics may show increased production of brain cells and showing down their destructions.
- These are drugs/supplements/nutraceuticals/functional foods that enhance one or more aspects of mental function.
- Use of prescription stimulants is prevalent among students facing examinations, e.g. dimethylamylamine, methylphenidate.
- Nootropics probably act by changing the levels of neurotransmitters, hormones or enzymes.
- They may also enhance the brain oxygen supply, energy supply or blood supply.
- There are nootropics available for providing sleep and rest and also for avoiding dizziness and to keep alert.

Q 3. What are the mechanisms of action of nootropic agents?

Principle mechanisms of action of nootropic agents:

1. Decreases malondialdehyde levels in brain and increases levels of antioxidant molecules such as glutathione and superoxide dismutase.
2. Interaction with dopamine D_2, serotonergic and GABA-B receptors.
3. Reduction of MAO-A and plasma corticosterone levels.
4. Reduces the concentration of noradrenaline and decreases turnover of central monoamines.
5. Inhibition of acetylcholinesterase activity in brain.
6. Increases content of lipids and phospholipids in brain.
7. Protects neurons against glutamate-induced toxicity.

H. CENTRALLY ACTING MUSCLE RELAXANTS

Q 1. Write a note on 'centrally acting muscle relaxants'.

Centrally Acting Muscle Relaxants

- Centrally acting muscle relaxants are used medically as adjuncts to rest, physical therapy and for the relief of discomfort associated with acute, painful musculoskeletal conditions.
- These agents are used in skeletal muscle spasms of local origin, multiple sclerosis, cerebral palsy, sprains, strains, fibrositis, rheumatoid spondylitis, arthritis.
- The muscle relaxant drugs can effectively reduce the rigidity of muscle without affecting the consciousness and normal voluntary movements of the muscles.
- Satisfactory muscle relaxation is valuable for operative procedure.
- These drugs are also useful for relieving convulsions of tetanus, strychnine poisoning drug-induced convulsions and various spastic disorders.

- These drugs act on muscle fibre or at neuromuscular junction or centrally in cerebrospinal axis.
- These drugs reduce muscle tone and cause paralysis.
- Centrally acting muscle relaxants act on selective areas in the CNS, thus effectively decreasing skeletal muscle tone and involuntary movements.
- Examples of centrally acting muscle relaxants:

1. Mephenesin
2. Methocarbamol
3. Chlorsoxazone
4. Metaxalone
5. Diazepam.

1. Mephenesin

- Mephenesin was the first drug found to cause muscle relaxation without producing unconsciousness.
- Mephenesin is an odourless, white crystalline powder, freely soluble in alcohol, chloroform and ether but insoluble in water.
- Mephenesin does not block the neuromuscular transmission.

Therapeutic uses/Indications

1. Mephenesin controls epileptic seizures within 30 seconds.
2. Mephenesin has a central sedative action and has been found to be useful in certain psychotic states.
3. Mephenesin antagonises strychnine convulsion.
4. Mephenesine provides muscular relaxation and relief from certain types of tremors as occurs in parkinsonism.
5. Mephenesin is used to obtain muscular relaxation in surgical anaesthesia.

Adverse Effects

- Damage to veins and haemolysis
- Weakness
- Nystagmus
- Double vision
- Drowsiness, nausea
- Respiratory depression.

Dosage

1. Mephenesin capsules : 250 and 500 mg capsules
2. Mephenesin injection : 10 mg per ml

Dose: 0.5–3 gm given slowly.

Brand name: Dolomed, Dolopar.

2. Methocarbamol

- It is a CNS depressant traditionally suggested for use in acute painful musculoskeletal conditions such as muscle tension and pains associated with anxiety states.
- The muscle relaxation property of this drug may be due to its sedative property.

Side Effects

- Drowsiness
- Dizziness
- Light headedness
- Blurred vision
- Black, blue or green discolouration of urine.

Therapeutic uses

1. To treat muscle spasm/pain.
2. Used in treatment of tetanus.
3. To treat muscle tension and pains associated with anxiety states.

Dosage

Mephenesin tablet : 1500 mg four times daily individed doses.

Brand names: Robaxin, ROBI-M, Robinax.

3. Chlorsoxazone

- Chlorsoxazone is a centrally acting muscle relaxant used to treat muscle spasm and the resulting pain or discomfort.
- It can also be administered for acute pain in general and for tension headache.
- It acts on the spinal cord by depressing reflexes.
- It also acts as muscle relaxant by virtue of its CNS depressant effect.
- The beneficial effect is due to sedative properties for the relief of muscle spasms.

Uses

1. As a centrally acting muscle relaxant.
2. To treat muscle spasm.
3. To reduce pain and discomfort.
4. To treat acute pain in general and tension headache.
5. For the relief of muscle spasms.

Adverse Effects

- Drowsiness
- Dizziness
- Nausea, vomiting
- Heartburn
- Constipation.

Dose: 750 mg 3–4 times daily orally.

Brand names: Lorzone, Remular-S.

I. OPIOID ANALGESICS

Q 1. Define and classify opioid analgesics/ narcotic analgesics with examples.

Opioid Analgesics

The drugs which produce narcosis along with analgesic effects are called opioid analgesics/narcotic analgesics/true analgesics.

Classification

a. Natural opium alkaloids, e.g. morphine, codeine.
b. Synthetic derivatives, e.g. heroin.
c. Synthetic morphine substitutes, e.g. pethidine, methadone.

Q 2. Write a note on morphine as opioid analgesic. OR Write a note on 'natural opium alkaloids' as opioid analgesics. OR Give the pharmacological actions, adverse effects, therapeutic uses, doses of the morphine.

Morphine

- Morphine is a principle alkaloid obtained from opium.
- Morphine belongs to phenanthrene class of alkaloids.
- Morphine was the first opioid analgesic discovered.
- Morphine has a biphasic effect on the CNS, i.e. it depresses the cerebrum while simultaneously depressing and stimulating the medulla.

Pharmacological Actions

a. **Antitussive:** Morphine acts as antitussive drug. It suppresses cough by depressing cough centres.
b. **Analgesic:** Morphine relieves severe pain, pain of trauma, with following mechanisms:
   i. It elevates the threshold and produces sleep.
   ii. It changes the emotional reaction to pain.
   iii. It elevates threshold of painful stimulus and relieves pain. Patient feels no pain.
c. **Action on eyes:** Morphine causes constriction of pupil (miosis). Morphine addicted persons have constricted eye pupils. Morphine produces a pinpoint constriction of the pupil.
d. **Action on respiratory system:** Morphine produces respiratory system depression. The depression of morphine on the respiration is central. Respiratory failure is the main cause of death. If patient dies of overdose of morphine.
e. **Action on urinary tract:** Morphine produces release of antidiuretic hormone (ADH) which results in decrease of urine output. The overall effect is of urinary retention.
f. **Action on central nervous system:** Morphine produces euphoria in presence of pain. In absence of pain, it produces dysphoria. Morphine when given in high doses produces sleep.
g. **Action on vomiting center:** Morphine stimulates the vomiting center, it produces vomiting due to stimulation of chemoreceptor trigger (CTZ). Tolerance develops to vomiting on prolonged used.
h. **Action on gastrointestinal tract:** Morphine decreases peristaltic movements. Secretions like hydrochloric acid, intestinal secretions are decreased. It

increases water absorption from intestinal tract so the faeces gets dried. These effects lead to constipation. Absorption of morphine from gastrointestinal tract is slow and incomplete. It is almost excreted in urine within 24 hours.

i. **Action on heart (cardiovascular system):** The morphine given in normal doses does not effect heart functioning or blood circulation. The higher doses of morphine cause hypotension.

j. **Action on biliary tract:** Morphine increases biliary pressure in man. Morphine evokes biliary spasm, due to its analgesic action.

k. **Action on smooth muscles:** It increases tone of uterus and decreases its peristalsis, produces constriction of bronchi.

Adverse Effects

1. Dryness of mouth
2. Constipation
3. Nausea, vomiting, headache
4. Mental clouding
5. Increased pressure in biliary tract
6. Skin rash, contact dermatitis
7. Hypotension
8. Tolerance
9. Dependence, addiction
10. It depresses foetal respiration if administered in pregnant women.

Therapeutic uses

1. It is used as a narcotic analgesic.
2. As a preanaesthetic medication.
3. For sedation and sleep.
4. To produce constipation or to treat diarrhoea.
5. It is a valuable drug in acute left ventricular failure.
6. It is most powerful analgesic agent for visceral pains.

Contraindications

Morphine is contraindicated in the following conditions:

- Acute respiratory depression
- Head injury
- Acute alcoholism
- Increased intracranial pressure.

Preparations and Doses

Preparation	*Dose*
1. Powdered opium IP	60–200 mg orally
2. Tincture opium IP	0.3–2 ml orally
3. Morphine hydrochloride tablet IP	8–20 mg orally
4. Morphine hydrochloride injection IP	8–20 mg subcutaneous or intramuscular injection

Q 3. Write a note on 'acute morphine poisoning'/acute opium poisoning.

Acute Morphine Poisoning/Acute Opium Poisoning

Acute morphine poisoning may occur due to clinical overdosage or accidental overingestion in an addict or from suicidal intention.

Signs and Symptoms

1. Dryness of mouth
2. Pinpoint pupil
3. Respiratory depression
4. Reduced body temperature
5. Reduced urinary output
6. Hypotension
7. Shock and coma
8. Constipation
9. Convulsions may occur in infants
10. Death is usually due to respiratory depression.

Treatments

A. Drug Treatment

The actions of morphine are antagonised by specific antagonists like naloxone and nalorphine.

These drugs significantly reverse morphine-induced respiratory depression.

a. **Naloxone:** It is usually preferred because of its specific antagonistic activity. It is given in the dose of 0.4–0.8 mg repeated every 10–15 minutes as required.

b. **Nalorphine:** It is antagonist of morphine and usually administered intravenously in the dose of 3–5 mg repeated within half an hour, if necessary.

B. Other Treatments

a. **Gastric lavage:** This is done by administration of emetic preparation to induce vomiting and withdrawal of gastric contents. For example, syrup of ipecac.

b. **Supportive treatments:** Such as maintenance of patient's airway, maintenance of BP, mechanical ventilation, nutrition by intravenous glucose saline and prevention of secondary infection.

c. **Anticonvulsants** like paraldehyde are used to reduce convulsions, if any.

Q 4. Write in brief about following opioid analgesics.

a. Codeine

- Methylmorphine is the chemical name for codeine.
- Codeine has a comparable pharmacological activity to morphine.
- In the body, it decomposes into methane and morphine.
- It is less potent and has a lower risk of addiction than morphine.
- It is less constipating than morphine.
- It depresses cough centre hence useful in the treatment of dry cough.
- It has synergistic effect with non-narcotic analgesic-like aspirin.

Adverse Effects

1. Respiratory depression
2. Drowsiness

Therapeutic uses

1. As an antitussive
2. To treat diarrhoea
3. As a opioid analgesic
4. As a sedative hypnotic
5. Also used in combination with aspirin.

Dose: 10–30 mg/day orally.

Brand names: Cosaka, Kefex, Glycodin.

b. Heroin

- Heroin is a diacetylmorphine.
- It is also known as dimorphine.
- Heroin is a semi-synthetic morphine derivative.
- It produces analgesic and respiratory depression.
- Analgesic effect of heroin is faster than morphine and it only lasts for 2–3 hours.

Adverse Effects

- Euphoria
- Drug addiction, drug dependance

c. Pethidine

- Pethidine is a synthetic narcotic analgesic.
- Pethidine has analgesic, sedative, spasmolytic and local anaesthetic action.
- Pethidine was discovered while looking for a spasmolytic with atropine-like effects.

Mechanism of Action

It depresses pain impulses by interacting with opioid receptors at the spinal cord level.

Adverse Effects

- Headache, sedation, drowsiness, dizziness.
- Euphoria
- Palpitation
- Blurred vision, miosis, diplopia, dryness of mouth.
- Nausea, vomiting, anorexia, constipation.
- Urinary retention, rash, urticaria.
- Respiratory depression.

Contraindications

- Hypersensitivity • Pregnancy and lactation • Respiratory depression.

Therapeutic uses

1. To relieve moderate to severe pains.
2. As a preanaesthetic medication.
3. As an analgesic during labour pains.
4. In treatment of morphine addiction as a substitute.
5. In the treatment of renal, biliary and intestinal colics.
6. In the treatment of pain in coronary thrombosis.

Q 5. What is euphoria? Name the drugs which produce this condition.

The condition of feeling of well-being is called euphoria. The drugs which produce euphoria are morphine, heroin, alcohol, etc.

Q 6. Give the difference between morphine and pethidine.

Morphine	*Pethidine*
• Absorption on oral administration is unpredictable. Administered by subcutaneous route	• Well absorbed on oral administration. Because of irritant nature, not administered by subcutaneous route
• Potent analgesic and narcotic	• Less potent analgesic
• Spasmogenic	• Spasmolytic
• Depress cough centre	• Does not depress cough centre
• Constrict pupil	• No effect
• Depress respiration in newborn hence, not useful to relieve labour pains	• Comparatively less depression of respiration, hence useful in labour pains

Q 7. Give the brand names, doses, route and major toxic effect of the following opioid analgesics.

Drug	*Brand name*	*Dose*	*Route*	*Major adverse effect*
1. Morphine	Morphitec	8–20 mg/day	Oral, SC, IM	Constipation, miosis
2. Codeine	Codicept, Glycodin	15–60 mg q.i.d.	Oral, SC, IM	Constipation, drowsiness
3. Pethidine	Meperidine, Demerol	300 mg/day	Oral, SC, IM	Sweating, dizziness, dryness of mouth

QUESTIONS: GIVE THE REASONS

Q 1. Why morphine causes constipation? OR Why tincture of opium is used in diarrhoea?

Morphine has spasmogenic action on smooth muscles of GIT.

i. It causes constriction of the sphincters and decreases in the peristaltic movements of GIT.
ii. This action of morphine results in stagnation of intestinal contents causing maximum absorption of water and drying of faecal matter.
iii. Morphine reduces sensitivity of intestinal walls to defaecation reflexes.
iv. The above actions of morphine cause constipation.
v. Tincture of opium contains morphine which possesses the constipating action. Hence, it is used in diarrhoea.

Q 2. In biliary colic, morphine is used along with atropine. Why?

Biliary colic means pains due to spasm of the biliary tract. To relieve the pains, analgesic drug morphine is used.

i. But morphine has spasmogenic action on the biliary tract which may aggravate the colicy pain.
ii. Hence, to relieve spasms, the antispasmodic drug-like atropine is used.
iii. These two drugs act synergistically in treatment of biliary colic.

Q 3. Morphine causes addiction. Why?

Morphine relieves severe type of pains associated with burns, fractures, parturition, terminal illness of cancer, myocardial infarction, etc.

i. When morphine is administered in absence of pain, it produces euphoria (false sense of well beingness).
ii. To experience the euphoria again and again individual develops habit.
iii. Tolerance to morphine is developed in the individual results in tendency to increase the dose to get the required euphoria.
iv. This eventually results in morphine addiction.

Q 4. Nalorphine (or naloxone) is used in morphine poisoning. Why?

Nalorphine is a rapidly acting drug, given parenterally to prevent the effects of morphine (opioids) poisoning.

i. It reverses the respiratory depressant, sedative hypotensive, analgesic and psychotomimetic effects of morphine.
ii. In the absence of morphine, it exhibits no pharmacological activity.
iii. Thus, nalorphine (or naloxone) acts as antagonist to morphine. Hence, nalorphine is used in morphine poisoning.

Q 5. A morphine addict is given methadone substitution therapy in hospital. Why?

Morphine is a narcotic analgesic having addiction liability.

i. Methadone is a synthetic compound having analgesic action equal to that of morphine.
ii. Methadone causes respiratory depression and constipation but it produces less euphoria and drowsiness than morphine.
iii. Methadone is slower in onset and longer in duration of action.
iv. Methadone suppresses the withdrawal syndrome in patients who are being withdrawn from morphine.
v. Methadone is effective orally and lacks hypnosis and addiction liability.
vi. Hence, a morphine addict is given methadone substitution therapy in hospital.

Q 6. Why morphine is not given in severe abdominal pain before diagnosis is made?

Morphine is narcotic analgesic which relieves pain without modifying the underlying pathological process.

i. It interferes with the diagnosis by masking pain and creates a false sense of security.
ii. It also induces vomiting.
iii. Its spasmogenic actions on the GIT and biliary tract are additional drawbacks.
iv. Therefore, morphine is not given in severe abdominal pain before diagnosis is made.

Q 7. Morphine is contraindicated in head injury. Why?

If morphine is administered in head injury, it further increases the intracranial pressure.

i. This masks the useful diagnostic and prognostic signs making management of the patient difficult.
ii. The effects of morphine such as respiratory depression, miosis and mental clouding also interfere with the diagnosis.
iii. Hence, morphine is contraindicated in head injury.

Q 8. Morphine is strictly contraindicated in children, old people and carrying women. Why?

Morphine if administered in children, may decrease the rate and depth of respiration because the systems in children are not properly developed to detoxify the drug.

i. In old people, morphine causes respiratory depression, bronchospasm and asthma.

ii. In carrying women, morphine may cross the placental barrier and depress the foetal respiration.
iii. Hence, it is strictly contraindicated in children, old people and carrying women.

Q 9. Pethidine is frequently employed as an obstetric analgesic. Why?

i. The advantage of pethidine as obstetric analgesic is its short duration which allows a better control on the level of drug.
ii. This reduces the risk of respiratory depression in the newborn.
iii. Pethidine causes relatively less respiratory depression in the newborn than does an equianalgesic dose of morphine.
iv. Pethidine lacks inhibitory action on uterine muscles. Pethidine does not suppress the cough reflex.
v. Hence, pethidine is frequently employed as an obstetric analgesic.

Objective Questions with Answers in Bold Letters

(Chapters: Antianxiety drugs, Antidepressants, Antipsychotics, Nootropics, Centrally acting muscle relaxants, Opioid analgesics).

1. Inability to sleep or lack of sleep means **insomnia.**
2. MAO inhibitors means **monoamine oxidase inhibitors.**
3. **Imipramine** is an example of tricyclic antidepressants.
4. Lithium carbonate is used as an **antianxiety drug.**
5. Librium is a popular brand name of **chlordiazepoxide.**
6. Meprobamate is an **anxiolytic drug.**
7. Depression is a **mental** illness, characterized by pathological changes in mood.
8. Nialamide and isocarboxazid are the examples of **MAO inhibitors.**
9. MAO inhibitors prevent oxidation of **catecholamine and histamine** in the brain.
10. **MAO inhibitors** potentiate the action of barbiturates, morphine and anaesthetics.
11. **Imipramine** is a dibenzazepine derivative used as a tricyclic antidepressants.
12. Imipramine is used to treat **enuresis.**
13. **Lithium carbonate** causes depletion of intraneural sodium and stabilises the neuronal membrane.
14. Lithium carbonate is contraindicated in **Addison's disease.**
15. Eating of **cheese** is forbidden in patients with MAO inhibitor therapy.
16. Schirophrenia means **'split mind' condition.**
17. Antidepressants are also known as mood **elevators/thymoleptics.**
18. Typical antipsychotic drugs act on dopaminergic system blocking the **dopamine type 2 (D_2) receptor.**
19. Chlorpromazine is a phenothiazine derivative used as **antipsychotic agent.**

20. Haloperidol is a **butyrophenone** derivative used as an antipsychotic agent.
21. Reserpine is a Rauwolfia alkaloid used as a **tranquillizer**.
22. **Chlorpromazine** is called 'Largactil'.
23. Antipsychotic action is due to competitive blockade of **dopaminergic receptors** in the limbic system.
24. Chlorpromazine **depresses CTZ** in the medulla and acts as a powerful antiemetic.
25. Chlorpromazine is adrug of choice in the treatment of **'schizophrenia'**.
26. Chlorpromazine is contraindicated in **pheochromocytoma**.
27. Reserpine is a principle alkaloid of '*Rauwolfia serpentina*' used in **snakebite**.
28. Reserpine produces depletion of **5-HT and catecholamines** from the brain and peripheral sites.
29. **Promethazine** is a drug used in the treatment of **motion sickness**.
30. Mania is a **bipolar** disorder.
31. Chlorpromazine is not effective in the vomiting of **motion sickness**.
32. Chlorpromazine produces **tranquillizing** effect.
33. **Reserpine** is not useful in immediate quietening or manic patients.
34. **Nootropics** are the supplementary drugs/substances.
35. Nootropics are called **'smart drugs'** that can boost brain performance.
36. Nootropics are sometimes called **'cognitive enhancers'**.
37. *Panax ginseng* and *Bacopa monnieri* are natural phytoconstituents used as **nootropics**.
38. Piracetam is a nootropic agent which is a derivative of **GABA (γ-amino-butyric acid)**.
39. Nootropics probably act by **changing the levels of neurotransmitters, hormones or enzymes**.
40. **Mephenesin, methacarbamol and chlorsoxazone** are central acting muscle relaxants.
41. **Mephenesin** was the first drug found to cause muscle relaxation without producing unconsciousness.
42. **Nystagmus** is an adverse effect of mephenesin.
43. Dolomed and Dolopar are the brand names of **mephenesin**.
44. The muscle relaxant properly of methocarbamol is due to its **sedative property**.
45. **Opioid analgesics** are also known as narcotic analgesics/true analgesics.
46. **Morphine** was the first opioid analgesic discovered.
47. Morphine has a **biphasic** effect.
48. Morphine produce **miosis (constriction of pupils)**.
49. **Morphine** decreases peristaltic movements and produce constipation.
50. Dryness of mouth and constipation are the major drawbacks of **morphine**.
51. **Naloxone and nalorphine** are the antidotes/antagonists used in the treatment of morphine poisoning/opium poisoning.
52. Methylmorphine is a chemical name of **codeine**.

53. The usual dose of codeine is **10–30 mg per day orally**.
54. Heroin is a **diacetylmorphine**.
55. Heroin is a **semi-synthetic** derivative of **morphine**.
56. **Pethidine** is a synthetic narcotic analgesic.
57. Pethidine depresses pain impulses by interacting with **opioid receptors** at the spinal cord level.
58. Constipation is the major adverse effect of **morphine**.
59. Morphine is contraindicated in **pregnancy and lactation**.
60. **Morphine** is used in the treatment of renal, biliary and intestinal colics.
61. The condition of feeling of well-being is called **euphoria**.
62. Glycodin is a popular brand name of **codeine**.
63. **Tincture of opium** is used in diarrhoea.
64. In biliary colic, morphine is used along with **atropine**.
65. Nalorphine or naloxone is used in **morphine poisoning**.
66. **Methadone** is a substitute of morphine.
67. **Morphine** is contraindicated in head injury.
68. Pethidine is used as an **obstetric analgesic**.
69. The dose of naloxone is **0.4–0.8 mg** repeated every 10–15 minutes as required.
70. Morphine stimulates **CTZ** and produces vomiting.

Chapter 5

Drugs Acting on Cardiovascular System

- Antihypertensive drugs
- Antiarrhythmic drugs
- Drugs used in congestive heart failure (CHF)
- Antianginal drugs
- Drugs used in atherosclerosis
- Drug therapy for shock

A. ANTIHYPERTENSIVE DRUGS

Q 1. What is hypertension? Define and classify antihypertensive drugs giving suitable examples.

Hypertension

- Hypertension is the abnormal elevation in blood pressure.
- Hypertension means high systemic blood pressure due to defect in the haemodynamic function.
- The WHO defined hypertension in adult as 'a systolic pressure equal to or greater than 160 mm Hg and a diastolic pressure equal to or greater than 95 mm Hg.

Types

a. **Primary hypertension (essential hypertension):** In this case the exact cause is not known. But there is generally narrowing of blood vessels. It may be benign hypertension or malignant hypertension.
b. **Secondary hypertension:** It may be caused due to secondary disorders like renal disorders, endocrine disorders or toxemia of pregnancy.

Antihypertensive Drugs

The drugs which reduce elevated blood pressure to normal level are called antihypertensive drugs. The drugs used in the treatment of hypertension are called antihypertensive drugs.

Classification

1. Drugs acting centrally, e.g. clonidine, methyldopa.
2. Drugs acting on autonomic ganglia, i.e. ganglion blocking agents, e.g. hexamethonium, mecamylamine, pempidine, trimethaphan.
3. Drugs acting on post-ganglionic sympathetic nerve endings.
   a. Adrenergic neuron blockers, e.g. guanethidine.
   b. Catecholamine depletors, e.g. reserpine.

4. Drugs acting on adrenergic receptors.
   a. α-Adrenergic blockers, e.g. phenoxybenzamine, phentolamine.
   b. β-Adrenergic blockers, e.g. propranolol.
5. Drugs acting directly on vascular smooth muscles, i.e. vasodilators, e.g. Hydralazine, diazoxide, minoxidil, sodium nitroprusside.
6. Drugs acting reflexely by stimulating baroreceptor, e.g. veratrum.
7. Drugs which block renin angiotensin aldosterone axis, e.g. saralsin, spironolactone, captopril, enalapril.
8. Oral diuretics, e.g. thiazides (hydrochlorthiazide).
9. Miscellaneous, e.g. MAO inhibitors (pargyline), nifedipine, sodium nitroprusside.

Q 2. Write a note on centrally acting antihypertensives (clonidine and methyldopa).

The centrally acting antihypertensives:

a. Clonidine

Pharmacological actions: Clonidine is a potent antihypertensive drug. When given IV, it produces a short hypertensive response followed by a prolonged hypotension. Hence, it is not suitable drug in hypertensive emergencies. The initial rise in blood pressure is because of its adrenergic agonist action. The major antihypertensive action of clonidine is central. The α-adrenergic receptors in the vasomotor centre are stimulated by clonidine. This inhibits peripheral sympathetic activity. Clonidine also reduces PRA (plasma renin activity). It causes decrease in cardiac output due to both, a decrease in stroke volume and bradycardia. It causes significant reduction in total peripheral resistance in standing position.

Adverse Reactions

It causes drowsiness and dryness of mouth due to central inhibition of salivation. Besides this vertigo, constipation, GIT disturbances and allergic reactions can also occur.

Therapeutic uses

i. **Antihypertensive**
ii. **In migraine:** Clonidine hydrochloride administered orally in the dose of 0.025 mg twice daily appears to be prophylatically useful in migraine patients.

b. Methyldopa

Pharmacological actions: It decreases heart rate. The fall in blood pressure is more in hypertensive than in normotensive subjects. The hypotensive effect is associated with reduction in cardiac output and in total peripheral resistance. Its hypotensive effect is enhanced by simultaneous use of thiazides.

Indication/uses: Hypertension in pregnancy.

Contraindications: Depression, active liver disease, pheochromocytoma, porphyria.

Dosage: Tablets of methyldopa 250 mg are available.

Hypertension in pregnancy: Initially 250 mg two to three times daily gradually increased to maximum 3 gm daily.

Q 3. Describe in brief 'ganglionic blocking agents' as antihypertensives.

Ganglionic Blocking Agents

This class includes the drugs: Hexamethonium, mecamylamine, pempidine, trimethaphan, etc.

Pharmacological Action

These drugs block the transmission of impulses in the sympathetic as well as parasympathetic ganglia. They do not prevent the release of ACh at ganglion but produce ganglionic blockade by occupying the receptor sites on the ganglion cells. This results in the reduction in the amount of noradrenaline released from postganglionic sympathetic nerve endings and this induces reduction in peripheral sympathetic tone and falls in blood pressure.

Adverse Reactions

1. Because of **parasympathetic blocked effect**, visual disturbances, mydriasis, cycloplegia, constipation, paralytic ileus and urinary retention are some adverse reactions.
2. **Sympathetic blockade:** Marked hypotension, disturbances in sexual function in male, sudden pulmonary oedema.
3. **Central actions:** Mental confusion tremors and seizures.
4. Tolerance.

Preparations

Pentolinium tartarate 10–40 mg tab.

Mecamylamine hydrochloride IP 2.5 mg tablet.

B. ANTIANGINAL DRUGS (VASODILATORS)

Q 1. What is angina pectoris? Mention the drugs used in treatment of angina pectoris.

Angina Pectoris

- Angina pectoris is a heart disease in which there is a paroxysmal pains in the chest, usually due to interference with the supply of oxygen to the heart muscle and precipitated by excitement.

- Angina pectoris refers to the chest pain towards left arm shoulder due to less supply or more demand of oxygen.
- Angina is due to imbalance between myocardial oxygen requirement and oxygen supply.

Signs and Symptoms: Chest pains, shortness of breath, sweating, fainting.

Drugs used in angina pectoris: Isosorbide dinitrate, glyceryl trinitrate, propranolol, verapamil, nifedipine, amlodipine, diltiazem.

Q 2. Define and classify antianginal drugs/vasodilators with examples.

Antianginals/Vasodilators

The drugs are used in the treatment of angina pectoris by dilating the blood vessels are called antianginals or vasodilators.

Classification

A. **On the basis of mode of action:**
   1. Nitrates, e.g. glyceryl trinitrate, isosorbide dinitrate.
   2. β-Blockers, e.g. propranolol, metoprolol, atenolol.
   3. Calcium channel blockers, e.g. verapamil, diltiazem, nifedipine, amlodipine.
   4. Potassium channel opener, e.g. nicorandil.

B. **Peripheral vasodilators**, e.g. tolazoline.

C. **Coronary vasodilators**, e.g. glyceryl trinitrate, ethyl nitrite, amyl nitrate.

Q 3. Write a note on 'drugs used in angina pectoris'. OR Explain glyceryl trinitrate/nitrite as an antianginal agent.

Angina Pectoris

Angina pectoris is a disorder resulting due to cardiac ischaemia. In this condition there is a compressing type of pain in the chest. Coronary vasodilators are useful in the treatment of angina pectoris.

Glyceryl Trinitrate/Nitrite

Organic nitrites are potent vasodilators and successfully used in therapy of angina pectoris for many years.

Mechanism of Action

- The effects of nitrates are mediated through the direct relaxant action on smooth muscles.
- Nitrates are believed to act by enhancing the vasodilator action of endothelium derived relaxing factor (EDRF) identified as nitrous oxide.
- Vasodilating organic nitrites are reduced to organic nitrites, which are then converted to nitric oxide.

- The action of nitrites begins after 2–3 minutes when chewed or held under tongue and action lasts for 2 hours.

Pharmacological Action of Glyceryl Trinitrate/Nitrite

1. Cardiovascular Action

- The post-arterial vascular bed is mainly affected by the action of nitrites.
- Arterioles dilate much more than bigger vessels.
- Vasodilation varies in different regions.
- Cutaneous vasodilation occurs on inhalation of a volatile nitrite, like amyl nitrite.
- In general blood pressure falls, the systolic more than the diastolic resulting in reduced pulse pressure.

2. Effect on the Heart

Increased coronary supply improves the nutrition of the myocardium thus anginal pain is relieved.

3. Action on Smooth Muscles

The nitrites produce relaxation of smooth muscles of bronchi, intestine, uterus, biliary tract and oesophagus.

4. Action on Haemoglobin

Nitrites convert blood haemoglobin to methemoglobin. Methemoglobin formed combines with the cyanides to form non-toxic cyanmethemoglobin. Thus, nitrites are useful in cyanide poisoning treatment.

Adverse Effects/Toxic Effects

1. Methemoglobinemia
2. Increased intraocular tension
3. Syncope
4. Hypertension
5. Headache, flushing of face, dizziness, fainting due to fall in blood pressure.
6. Tolerance

Contraindications

1. In severe anemia
2. In glaucoma
3. In idiosyncrasy.

Therapeutic uses

1. In prophylaxis and treatment of angina pectoris.
2. In post-myocardial infarction.
3. In coronary insufficiency.

4. In acute left ventricular failure (LVF).
5. To treat unstable angina.
6. To treat congestive heart failure.
7. For the relief of coronary artery spasm.
8. To treat acute cardiopulmonary edema.
9. To treat postoperative hypertension.

Preparations and Doses

1. Sodium nitrite	: 0.3–0.5 gm	: By IV route
2. Amyl nitrite	: 0.3 ml of drug	: Inhalation
3. Glyceryl trinitrate	: 0.3–0.6 mg every 8–12 hours	: Sublingual
4. Octyl nitrite	: 0.2 ml of drug	: Inhalation
5. Isosorbide dinitrate	: 5–10 mg	: Sublingually

Q 4. Write a note on calcium channel blockers, as an antianginal drug.

The drugs which block the calcium entry into the myocardium are called calcium channel blockers.

Calcium is necessary for the excitation and contraction in both skeletal and smooth muscle. The contractility of skeletal, cardiac and vascular muscle is highly dependant on the extracellular calcium concentration.

The calcium channel blockers act by interfering with calcium entry into the myocardium and thus decreasing the availability of intracellular Ca^{++}. Due to this, there is a decrease in myocardial contractility.

Calcium channel blockers are useful in angina pectoris because of following reasons:

i. Decrease in myocardial contractility
ii. Decrease in oxygen consumption
iii. Decrease in preload to heart
iv. Increase in coronary blood flow due to dilation of coronary blood vessels.

- Preparations
  1. Verapamil tablet IP

     Dose: 240–480 mg/day orally.

     Trade name: Cardilox
  2. Nifedipine tablet IP

     Dose: 10 mg 8 hourly

     Trade name: Calciguard.

C. ANTIARRHYTHMIC DRUGS

Q 1. What is arrhythmia/cardiac arrhythmia? Define and classify anti-arrhythmic agents.

Arrhythmia/Cardiac Arrhythmia

It means disturbance in cardiac rhythm or heart beat. Arrhythmia can be caused by disturbance in conduction of impulse throughout the myocardium of heart.

Types

1. Tachycardia: Heart rate above 100 beats per minute.
2. Bradycardia: Heart rate lower than 60 beats per minute.
3. Atrial fibrillation.
4. Atrial flutter.
5. Ventricular flutter.
6. Extra systole.

Symptoms

- Fatigue,
- Dizziness
- Fainting
- Rapid heart beat
- Shortness of breath
- Chest pain
- Anxiety

Antiarrhythmic Agents

The drugs which are used in the treatment of cardiac arrhythmia are called antiarrhythmic agents.

Classification

1. Drugs that depress the myocardium.
   a. Electrophysiologically always depressent, e.g. quinidine, procainamide, potassium.
   b. Electrophysiologically partial depressent, e.g. lignocaine, phenytoin.
2. Drugs acting through autonomic nervous system.
   a. Sympatholytics—β-blockers, e.g. propranolol, practolol.
   b. Cholinergic, e.g. edrophonium.

Mechanism of Action

1. Slowing of diastolic depolarisation: Decrease in enhanced automaticity of ectopic focci slows conduction velocity.
2. Elevation of threshold potential of myocardiac cells.
3. Increase in diastolic intracellular negativity which prolongs the spontaneous diastolic depolarisation.
4. Slowing of K^+ efflux from myocardial cells, i.e. re-entry mechanism is blocked.

Q 2. Write a note on 'quinidine' and 'procainamide' as an antiarrhythmic agent.

a. Quinidine

It is an alkaloid obtained from Cinchona bark.

Pharmacological Actions

1. Automaticity: Quinidine depresses the automaticity.
2. Excitability: Quinidine depresses excitability of cardiac tissue.
3. Refractory period: Quinidine prolongs the refractory period.
4. Conduction velocity: Quinidine decreases conduction velocity in all cardiac tissues.
5. AV conduction: Quinidine depresses the myocardial contractility.

Adverse Effects

1. Cardiac toxicity: Bradycardia, conduction block, ventricular fibrillation.
2. Embolic phenomenon: Formation of emboli or thrombus into the circulation.
3. Hypotension: Quinidine produces hypotension in larger doses.
4. Cinchonism.

- **Preparation:** Quinidine sulphate tablet or capsule IP.

  Dose: 200–400 mg every 6 hours.
- **Therapeutic uses (indications):** Quinidine is indicated in the following conditions:

1. Atrial fibrillation
2. Atrial flutter
3. Ventricular fibrillation
4. Ventricular flutter.

Contraindications: In complete heart block.

b. Procainamide

Procainamide is effective both orally as well as by injection route. It is free from toxic effects on central nervous system. Its local anaesthetic properties are similar to procaine.

Pharmacological Actions

- Procainamide depresses excitability of cardiac tissue, depresses myocardial contractility and conduction velocity in all cardiac tissues.
- Blood pressure which causes hypotension.

Adverse Reactions

Hypotension and psychosis may develop. Anorexia, nausea, vomiting, cardiotoxicity such as bradycardia, conduction block, ventricular fibrillation.

Therapeutic uses

It is used in the treatment of:

- Atrial and nodal premature beats
- Paroxysmal atrial tachycardia
- Ventricular premature beats
- Ventricular tachycardia
- Useful in patients in whom quinidine produces cinchonism.

Contraindications

1. In heart block
2. In heart failure
3. In hypotension.

Dosage

Procainamide tablet : 1 gm followed by 50 mg/kg/day orally in divided doses

D. DRUGS USED IN ATHEROSCLEROSIS

Q 1. What do you mean by atherosclerosis? Classify the drugs used in atherosclerosis (antiatherosclerotic/antihyperlipidemic drugs).

Atherosclerosis

- It means hardening of blood vessels due to hyperlipidaemia.
- In this condition, there is a deposition of lipid/fatty material in the inner walls of arteries. This may lead to coronary thrombosis and myocardial infarction.
- The deposition of fatty material in the walls of artery leads to thickening of artery which causes resistance in blood circulation and thus, increases blood pressure.
- Cholesterol is one of the important constituents which is a causative factor for atherosclerosis.
- In atherosclerosis there may be a patch generation developed in the 'tunica media' of large and medium sized arteries.
- This patch consists of accumulation of cholesterol compounds, excess of smooth muscles and fibroelastic cells.
- When these 'plaques' grow, they spread along the walls of artery forming swelling which may produce resistance in blood circulation. This condition is called atherosclerosis.
- Atherosclerosis is regarded as a disorder in lipid metabolism.
- Hyperlipidaemia is a major cause of atherosclerosis and associated conditions are coronary heart disease (CHD), ischaemic cerebrovascular disease and peripheral vascular disease.

Classification of antiatherosclerotic/antihyperlipidemic drugs (lipid lowering agents):

1. **Drugs reducing biosynthesis of cholesterol (statins):** Atorvastatin, simvastatin, pravastatin, rosuvastatin.
2. **Bile-acid binding resins:** Cholestyramine, betasitosterol.
3. **Fibric acid derivatives:** Clofibrate, fenofibrate.
4. **Cholesterol absorption inhibitors:** Ezetimibe.
5. **Miscellaneous agents:** Nicotinic acid, neomycin.

Dosage of antisclerotic/antihyperlipidemic/lipid lowering agents:

1. Clofibrate tablet	: 2 gm daily in divided doses	: Atromid-S
2. Nicotinic acid tablet	: 1.5–8 gm/day	: Niacin
3. Lovastatin tablet	: 20–40 mg strengths	: Mevacor

E. DRUGS USED IN CONGESTIVE HEART FAILURE (CHF)

Q 1. What is CHF? Define cardiotonics with examples. Describe the drugs used in CHF. OR Write a note on digitalis/digoxin/cardiac glycosides as a cardiotonics. OR Give the pharmacological actions, adverse effects, therapeutic uses, contraindications of digitalis/digoxin.

Congestive Heart Failure (CHF)/(CCF)

- CHF is a pathophysiologic state in which the heart is unable to pump the blood at a rate of fulfill the requirements of body tissues.
- The force of contraction of heart is weak and thus ventricles cannot completely eject out the blood.
- This results in congestion of venous blood in different parts of the body causing edema, increased venous pressure, difficulty in respiration (dyspnoea) and weakness.
- The major organs affected due to CHF are liver, spleen and kidneys.
- CHF is also known as congestive cardiac failure or low output failure.
- Drugs used in CHF/CCF are:
  a. Cardiac glycosides, e.g. digitalis, strophanthus, squill.
  b. Vasodilators, e.g. glyceryl trinitrate.
  c. Diuretics, e.g. chlorthiazide, mersalyl, spironolactone.

Cardiotonics

The drugs which increase the activity of heart are called cardiotonics.

Digitalis

Digitalis is the most commonly employed cardiac glycoside, used as a cardiotonic drug.

Mechanism of Action

The Ca^{2+} is essential for myocardial contractility. Digitalis inhibits sodium-potassium pump and ↑ ses entry of Na^+ into the cell. This extracellular Na^+ exchanges for the intracellular K^+. Due to exchange between Na^+ and K^+, the intracellular Ca^{2+} concentration ↑ ses. Digitalis also ↑ ses the Ca^{2+} stores in the cells and due to Ca^{2+}, ↑ ses myocardial contractility.

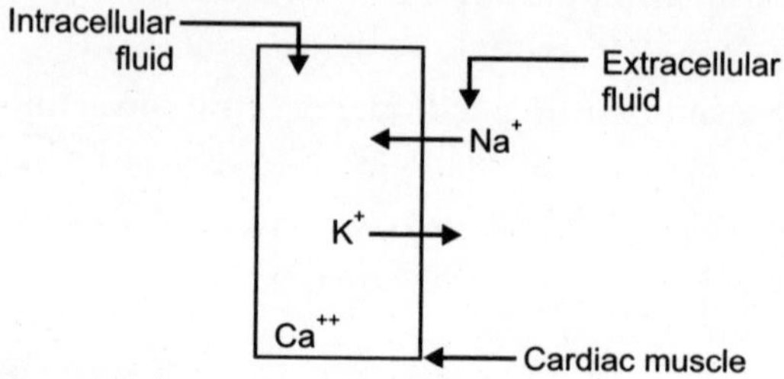

Pharmacological Actions

1. **Myocardial contractility:** Digitalis increases the force of systolic contraction of the heart muscles.
2. **Heart rate:** Digitalis produces decrease in heart rate by vagus stimulation.
3. **Conduction velocity:** Digitalis increases conduction velocity.
4. **Automaticity:** Digitalis increases the automaticity of ventricular muscles.
5. **BP:** Digitalis increases the mean arterial pressure.
6. **Refractory period:** Digitalis prolongs the functional refractory period of AV node.
7. **Digitalis and calcium:** Calcium ions increase the force of contraction of heart. Excessive Ca^{2+} ion concentration leads to cardiac arrest in systole. Digitalis acts synergistically with calcium. Hence, digitalis toxicity can be enhanced by calcium.

Adverse Effects

1. **GIT toxicity:** Anorexia, vomiting, diarrhoea.
2. **Cardiac toxicity:** Cardiac arrhythmia, ventricular tachycardia, ventricular fibrillation.
3. Hypokalemia (↑ se K^+ level in blood).
4. **Neurological toxicity:** Headache, visual disturbances like appearance of dancing and flickering dots and disturbance of colour vision.
5. **Miscellaneous toxicity:** Skin rash, digitalis can cross placental barrier and may lead to premature delivery.

Preparation and dose: Digoxin tablets IP

Dose: 0.25 mg once or twice daily.

Trade name: Lanoxin.

Therapeutic uses (Indications)

Digitalis is indicated in:

1. Congestive heart failure
2. Left ventricular failure
3. Atrial fibrillation
4. Atrial flutter

Contraindications

1. In hypersensitivity
2. In ventricular tachycardia
3. In AV block
4. In hypokalemia
5. In renal disease

F. DRUG THERAPY FOR SHOCK

Q 1. What do you mean by shock? Explain various drug therapies for shock.

Shock

- Shock is rapidly developing syndrome caused by inadequate capillary perfusion of vital tissues.
- Shock is a clinical syndrome characterized by collapse of peripheral circulation under various conditions.
- Shock is a state of acute circulatory failure in which the cardiac output is unable to maintain tissue perfusion for nutrition, oxygenation and waste disposal.
- Shock is immediately life-threatening emergency situation, as delivery of oxygen and nutrients to body organ is severely impaired.
- Shock is seen in conditions like heart attacks and strokes.

Reasons/Causes

- Multiple fractures
- Reactions to fear of fight or hearing bad news
- Internal tissue damage
- Haemorrhage
- Serious head injury
- Chest injury
- Abdominal injury
- Poisoning
- Disturbances in CVS function, etc.

Types

1. **Neurogenic shock:** It is due to spinal cord injury.
2. **Bacteremic shock:** It is due to severe infections.
3. **Haemo-obstructive shock:** It is due to blockade of a main blood vessels.

4. **Hypovolemic shock:** It is due to dehydration or severe blood loss. The dehydration may be due to intestinal obstruction, diarrhoea, vomiting, cholera or severe burns.
5. **Cardiogenic shock:** It may be due to extensive myocardial infarction, severe arrhythmia, obstruction to cardiac output, etc.
6. **Anaphylactic shock:**

- Anaphylactic shock is a rare but severe allergic reaction.
- Anaphylaxis causes the immune system to release a flood of chemicals that can cause shock which includes a sudden slowing of blood pressure, narrowing of airways and blocking breathing.
- The signs and symptoms of anaphylactic shock include:
  - A rapid, weak pulse
  - Nausea and vomiting
  - Feeling of warmth
  - A skin rash
  - Paleness
  - Hypotension.
- The antibiotics like penicillins may cause anaphylactic shock.
- Anaphylactic shock requires prompt treatment of possible laryngeal edema, bronchospasm and hypotension.

Treatment of Anaphylactic Shock

1. **Sympathomimetics (adrenergics):** Adrenaline injection 1 in 1000 by intramuscular route. Adults: 500 μg, may be repeated if necessary at 5 minutes intervals, depending on blood pressure, pulse and respiratory function.
2. **Vital functions:** Maintain an open airway give oxygen by mask, restore blood pressure.
3. **Antihistamine:** Chlorpheniramine by IV injection over 1 minute. Adult: 10–20 mg repeated if necessary.
4. **Corticosteroids:** Hydrocortisone by IV injection. Adult: 100–300 mg.
5. **Intravenous fluids:** Infusion sodium chloride (0.5–1 L during first hour).
6. If patient shows asthma-like symptoms give salbutamol 2.5–5 mg by nebulization.

QUESTIONS: GIVE THE REASONS

Q 1. Why digitalis is called 'cardiotonic'?

i. Digitalis has direct action on the myocardium of heart.
ii. It increases the force of systolic contraction.
iii. This leads to complete ventricular emptying with increase in stroke output.
iv. The duration of systole is decreased allowing greater time for ventricular filling and heart rest.

v. The diastolic size of the heart is reduced. Hence, oxygen expenditure for given work output is reduced and thus the working capacity of the heart is increased.

vi. Digitalis does not increase energy production by the cardiac muscle but improves its energy utilisation (i.e. conversion of chemical energy into mechanical energy).

vii. The digitalised heart thus can do same work with less energy or more work with same energy expenditure.

Therefore, digitalis is called cardiotonic.

Q 2. Why digitalis controls ventricular rate in atrial fibrillation?

i. Digitalis is used in the treatment of CCF.

ii. Digitalis shows predominant vagal effect on atrial muscles to shorten the refractory period.

iii. It reduces the ventricular rate in spite of the increased number of impulses reaching the conducting tissue.

iv. Digitalis by its vagal and direct action on AV node, prolong the refractory period.

v. Thus, digitalis depresses the conduction across the AV bundle and AV node and protects the ventricles from too rapid atrial impulses. Hence, digitalis controls ventricular rate in atrial fibrillation and improves circulation.

Q 3. Why patient on digitalis therapy is given potassium supplement?

i. Digitalis is used in the treatment of congestive cardiac failure (CCF).

ii. In CCF, because of increased sodium retention and disturbed aldosterone mechanism there is some degree of potassium loss.

iii. The restriction of sodium intake and prolonged diuretic therapy further increases the potassium loss.

iv. The excessive potassium loss may precipitate digitalis cardiotoxicity.

v. Therefore to reduce the digitalis toxicity, potassium supplement is given along with it.

Q 4. Why toxicity of digitalis is increased by chlorthiazide?

i. Chlorthiazide is a diuretic drug.

ii. Thiazides depress sodium transport in the cortical diluting segment of nephron just proximal to the point of Na–K exchange.

iii. Thiazides also increase potassium excretion to a considerable extent.

iv. In the treatment of congestive cardiac failure with digitalis, there is already excess potassium loss (due to excess sodium retention causing edema), i.e. hypokalemia.

v. Hence, if chlorthiazide diuretics are administered in patients on digitalis therapy then these increases the toxicity of digitalis.

Q 5. Why procainamide is preferred over procaine in management of cardiac arrhythmia?

i. Procainamide is more stable in the body, i.e. it has sufficient duration of action, when administered orally or parenterally.

ii. Procainamide does not stimulate CNS when administered intravenously.

iii. Whereas the procaine is not effective orally and has short duration of action.

iv. Procaine stimulates the CNS when administered intravenously.

v. Thus, procainamide differs from procaine due to replacement of the ester linkage by an amide linkage.

vi. Therefore, procainamide is preferred over procaine in the management of cardiac arrhythmias.

Objective Questions with Answers in Bold Letters

1. The drugs which increase the activity of heart are called **cardiotonics**.
2. **Clofibrate** is used as a lipid lowering agent.
3. The **calcium** is essential for myocardial contractility.
4. Digitalis inhibits **sodium-potassium pump**.
5. **Hypokalemia** is a adverse effect of digitalis.
6. **Lanoxin** is a popular brand name of digoxin.
7. Digitalis is indicated in **congestive heart failure (CHF)**.
8. Verapamil and nifedipine are **calcium channel blockers**.
9. Quinidine is used as an **antianginal drug**.
10. **Quinidine** depresses the automaticity and excitability of cardiac tissue.
11. Glyceryl trinitrate is an **antianginal drug**.
12. **Calciguard** is a popular brand name of nifedipine.
13. **Guanethidine** is an adrenergic neurone blocker.
14. **α-Methyldopa** is a centrally acting antihypertensive.
15. Clofibrate is a drug used in **atherosclerosis**.
16. **Digitalis** is a Na^+, K^+ ATPase inhibitor.
17. Methyldopa produces **postural hypotension**.
18. **Quinidine** is contraindicated in congestive heart failure.
19. Pheochromocytoma is an adverse effect of **propranolol**.
20. Digitalis is called **cardiotonic**.

21. The patient on digitalis therapy is given a potassium supplement to prevent **hypokalemia**.
22. **Angina pectoris** is a disease characterized by pains in the chest.
23. **Arrhythmia** is the disturbance or irregularity in cardiac rhythm.
24. Amyl nitrite is used in **cyanide poisoning**.
25. Glyceryl trinitrate is given by **sublingual route**.
26. Enalapril, ramipril and captopril are the **angiotensin-converting enzyme inhibitors**.
27. Valsartan and losartan are **angiotensin blockers**.
28. Verapamil produces **coronary vasodilation**.
29. The drug of choice in myocardial infarction is **streptokinase**.
30. The maintenance dose of digoxin in adult is **0.25–1.5 mg orally**.
31. **Digitalis** crosses placental barrier and may lead to premature delivery.
32. Glyceryl trinitrate is mainly used in the treatment of **angina pectoris**.
33. Quinidine and procainamide act as an **antiarrhythmic agent**.
34. Digitalis acts on heart by **increasing the force of contraction**.
35. The plasma half life of digoxin is **36 hours**.
36. Quinidine is contraindicated in **atrial fibrillation**.
37. Amyl nitrite is usually administered by **inhalation**.
38. Digitalis toxicity can be treated by **potassium supplement**.
39. The common name for digitalis is **fox glove**.
40. **Diplopia and blurred vision** are the adverse effects of digitalis on eye.

Chapter 6

Drugs Acting on Blood and Blood Forming Organs

- Haematinics
- Antiplatelet agents
- Anticoagulants
- Thrombolytic/fibrinolytic drugs

A. HAEMATINICS

Q 1. What is anaemia? Classify/give types of anaemia.

Anaemia

- A decrease in oxygen carrying capacity of blood is called anaemia.
- Anaemia means decrease in number of RBCs in the blood or decrease in percentage of haemoglobin in the blood.
- Erythropoiesis is the process of formation of erythrocytes in the red bone marrow.
- The deficiency of dietary factors such as iron, folic acid, vitamin B_{12}, etc. disturbs normal erythropoiesis resulting into anaemia.

Causes

1. Excess of blood loss (haemorrhage).
2. Failure of function of red bone marrow to produce RBCs.
3. Destruction of RBCs by haemolysis.
4. Deficiency of dietary factors such as iron, folic acid, vitamin B_{12}, vitamin C, etc.
5. Loss of blood due to menorrhagia.
6. Aplasia or hypoplasia of bone marrow produces aplastic and hypoplastic anaemia.
7. Due to infection or liver diseases.

Classification/Types

Morphologically anaemia can be classified as:

1. Microcytic hypocromic anaemia where size of red blood cells (RBCs) is smaller than normal and amount of haemoglobin is less than normal.
2. Microcytic anaemia where size of RBCs is smaller than normal.
3. Macrocytic anaemia where size of RBCs is larger than normal.

4. Normocytic normocromic anaemia where only number of RBCs is less.
5. Normocytic hypocromic anaemia.
6. Macrocytic hypocromic anaemia is dimorphic anaemia.
7. Haemolytic anaemia due to destruction of RBCs.
8. Iron deficiency anaemia due to loss of iron by haemorrhage.
9. Megaloblastic anaemia due to deficiency of vitamin B_{12}.
10. Sickle cell anaemia where shaped of RBC changes.
11. Pernicious anaemia due to lack of instrinsic factor.

Haematinics

The drugs which increase the number of RBCs and the amount of haemoglobin level in the blood are called haematinics.

Haematinics are used for the treatment of anaemia. Examples:

i. Iron
ii. Folic acid
iii. Vitamin B_{12}
iv. Ferrous sulphate
v. Liver extract
vi. Ferrous gluconate

Treatments

1. In macrocytic anaemia due to any cause, liver extract, vitamin B_{12}, folic acid, each alone or in any combination are used. But in pernicious anaemia vitamin B_{12} is specific.
2. In hypocromic anaemias and in microcytic anaemia, iron is specific.
3. In dimorphic anaemia treatment with combination of haemopoietic factors (iron being a constant factor), the combination such as iron and liver extract, iron, folic acid and vitamin B_{12}, etc. are used.
4. In very severe anaemia, e.g. haemoglobin 20% or below, due to any cause; blood transfusion is necessary.
5. In all cases of anaemia side by side with the treatment of anaemia the etiological treatment should also be given.

Q 2. Write a note on 'iron preparations' as haematinics.

Iron

- Iron is an essential factor for normal haemopoiesis.
- Iron is found especially in liver, egg-yolk, spinach and peas.
- It has a medicinal value in the treatment of anaemia.
- Iron requirements are greatly increased during growth, pregnancy, menstruation and haemorrhage condition.

- In iron deficiency anaemia, the iron requirement is up to 60 mg or more per day.
- Oral dose of iron is 100–200 mg daily.

Side Effects

i. GIT irritation
ii. Nausea
iii. Epigastric pains
iv. Diarrhoea
v. Constipation
vi. Black and red terry stools
vii. Discolouration of teeth

Uses

i. In iron deficiency anaemia
ii. In haemorrhage condition
iii. Iron deficiency in pregnancy.

Preparations

i. Ferrous sulphate dried : 200–300 mg daily
ii. Ferrous gluconate : 1.2–1.8 mg in divided doses daily
iii. Ferrous fumarate : 200–400 mg in divided doses
iv. Ferrous succinate : 200–400 mg in divided daily doses
v. Colloidal iron : 200–400 daily
vi. Ferrous ammonium citrate : 200–400 daily
vii. Sodium iron edetate : 150 mg daily
viii. Iron dextran injection (50 mg/ml) : 1 ml by IM (lmferon)
ix. Iron sorbitol injection (50 mg/ml) : 1.5 mg/kg IM (Jectofer)

Contraindications

- Hypersensitivity
- Cirrhosis of liver
- Peptic ulcer disease.

Q 3. What is iron poisoning (acute iron intoxication)? Give its signs, symptoms and treatment.

Iron Poisoning (Acute Iron Intoxication)

Iron poisoning may result from ingestion of more than 50 gm of iron.

Signs and Symptoms

i. Abdominal pain
ii. Vomiting
iii. Acidosis
iv. Cardiovascular collapse
v. Coma and finally death
vi. Gastric haemorrhage
vii. Circulatory collapse

Treatment

i. Gastric lavage with 1% sodium bicarbonate.
ii. IV administration desferroxamine (antidote).

iii. Fluid and electrolyte replacement.

Q 4. Write a note on 'cyanocobalamin and folic acid' as haematinics.

1. Cyanocobalamin (Vitamin B_{12})

- Cyanocobalamin is synthesized by microorganisms in intestines of animal, in soil and water.
- The vegetarians get vitamin B_{12} from milk, milk products, nodulated root vegetables and legumes.
- The non-vegetarians get vitamin B_{12} from food like liver, kidney, fish eggs and meat muscles.
- Vitamin B_{12} is made-up of a porphyrin-like ring with a central cobalt atom attached to a nucleotide.
- The ultimate source of vitamin B_{12} is from microbial synthesis.
- Vitamin B_{12} is a water-so0luble vitamin and occurs as thermostable red crystals.
- It is also called antipernicious anaemia vitamin.
- Vitamin B_{12} acts as a co-enzyme in the synthesis of DNA and is also essential for various metabolisms in the body.
- The daily requirement of vitamin B_{12} in adult is 1 mg/day and in children are 0.2–1 mg/day.

Dosage

1. Cyanocobalamin injection IP : 100 mg/ml
2. Cyanocobalamin injection : 100, 500, 1000 mg/ml
3. Hydroxycobalamin injection : 1 mg/ml.

Uses

1. To treat pernicious anaemia
2. To treat haemolytic anaemia
3. To treat microcytic anaemia
4. It helps in maturation of RBCs
5. It helps in providing energy to central nervous system.

Adverse Effects

- Skin rash
- Pain at the site of injection
- Pulmonary edema
- Hypokalemia
- Flushing
- Anaphylactic shock
- Optic nerve atrophy
- Diarrhoea

2. Folic Acid

- It is also known as folacin/vitamin M/bacterial growth factor.
- It has been named folic acid because it is commonly found in green leaves,

liver, yeast, eggs, meat and dairy foods.
- Mitchell in 1941 isolated folic acid from spinach.
- Folic acid plays a role in the biosynthesis of purines and pyrimidines, i.e. DNA.

Dosage

Folic acid tablet : 5–20 mg orally

Side Effects

Flushing, bronchospasm

Contraindications

- Hypersensitivity
- Uncorrected pernicious anaemia
- Vitamin B_{12} deficiency anaemia

Therapeutic uses

Folic acid is used to treat:

i. Nutritional megaloblastic anaemia
ii. Anaemia due to impaired absorption
iii. Anaemia due to impaired utilization
iv. Used in synthesis of DNA
v. Useful for normal production of RBCs.

B. ANTICOAGULANTS

Q 1. Define and classify anticoagulants with examples. Write a note on 'heparin'.

Anticoagulants

The drugs which prevent coagulation of blood are called anticoagulants.

Classification

i. *In vivo* anticoagulants
   a. Rapid-acting (parenteral), e.g. heparin and derivatives.
   b. Slow-acting (oral), e.g. warfarin, phenindione, dicoumarol.
ii. *In vitro* anticoagulants, e.g. oxalic acid, sodium citrate.

Heparin

- Heparin is a mucopolysaccharide obtained from ox lung or intestinal mucosa of pig or sheep.
- It is a complex mucopolysaccharide with a large number of sulphate groups.
- Heparin acts *in vivo* and *in vitro* to prolong the clotting time.
- Heparin is not effective orally and should be given intravenously where

it acts almost at once to last for 4–6 hours.

Mechanism of Action

Heparin inhibits the activity of activated factor X, thus, inhibiting the formation of thrombin from prothrombin and fibrin from fibrinogen.

Adverse Effects (Toxicity of Heparin)

1. Bleeding
2. Alopecia
3. Allergic and anaphylactic reactions
4. Osteoporosis
5. Thrombocytopenia.

Therapeutic uses

1. As an anticoagulant in transfusion and dialysis procedure.
2. Treatment and prophylaxis of deep vein thrombosis, open heart surgery.
3. In pulmonary embolism
4. In myocardial infarction
5. To treat arterial and venous thrombosis

Contraindications

- Hypersensitivity
- Bleeding disorder (haemophilia)
- Thrombocytopenia
- Peptic ulcer

Dosage

Heparin sodium 1000 units/ml injection.

Q 2. Write a note on 'oral anticoagulants'.

Oral Anticoagulants

The drugs which are effective by oral route as anticoagulant are known as oral anticoagulants.

They take about 36–48 hours for anticoagulant effect to develop. Hence, called oral anticoagulants.

Oral anticoagulants act by competitively antagonising the actions of vitamin K as they have structural similarities, e.g. warfarin, acenocoumarin.

Warfarin

It is readily and completely absorbed by oral route. It is extensively bound to plasma albumin and, therefore, it has relatively long plasma half-life.

Side Effects

i. Haemorrhage, haematuria, urticaria
ii. Anorexia, nausea, vomiting, diarrhoea.

Therapeutic uses

i. In treatment of venous thrombosis and pulmonary embolism.
ii. In myocardial infarction.
iii. In rheumatic heart disease.
iv. In artificial heart valve to prevent emboli.

Preparations

i. Warfarin sodium tablet : 5 mg twice daily (Uniwarfin)
ii. Acenocoumarin tablet : 15 to 20 mg/day orally (Acitrom, Sintro).

Contraindications

- Hypersensitivity
- Pregnancy
- Lactation
- Peptic ulcer.

C. ANTIPLATELET AGENTS

Q 1. What are antiplatelet agents? Classify them. OR Write a note on 'antiplatelet agents'.

Antiplatelet Agents

Antiplatelet agents are the drugs which prevent thrombus formation by decreasing platelet aggregation.

- Anticoagulants, antiplatelet drugs, thrombolytics are together referred as antithrombotic drugs.
- Antiplatelet drugs (antiaggregates, antithrombotics) are also known as platelet agglutination inhibitors. Antiplatelet agents are oftenly known as blood thinners.

Classification

a. **Arachidonic acid pathway inhibitors**, e.g. aspirin.
b. **ADP pathway inhibitors**, e.g. clopidogrel, ticlopidine.
c. **Phosphodiesterase inhibitors**, e.g. dipyridamole.
d. **Glycoprotein llb/llla inhibitors**, e.g. abciximab, eptifibatide.

1. Acetylsalicylic Acid (Aspirin)

In the initial management of the acute attack of myocardial infarction 150–300 mg by mouth (preferably chewable or dispersible tablet) is given immediately for its antiplatelet effect.

Therapeutic uses/Indications

Prophylaxis of cerebrovascular disease or myocardial infarction, pyrexia, pain, inflammation and migraine.

Contraindications

Hypersensitivity to acetylsalicylic acid or any other NSAIDs, active peptic ulceration, hemophilia and other bleeding disorders.

Dosage

For prophylaxis of cerebrovascular disease or myocardial infarction by mouth 75–100 mg daily.

2. Clopidogrel

The active metabolite of clopidogrel selectively inhibits the binding of ADP (adenosine diphosphate) to its platelet P2Y12 receptor and the subsequent ADP-mediated activation of the glycoprotein complex, thereby inhibiting platelet aggregation. The combination of aspirin and clopidogrel reduces the risk of major ischaemic events compared with aspirin alone.

Therapeutic uses/Indications

1. Coronary artery disease: In myocardial infarction, aspirin is used immediately after thrombolytic therapy.
2. Cerebrovascular disease
3. Peripheral artery disease
4. Heart attack or stroke
5. Acute coronary syndrome

Dosage

Oral tablets of 75 mg and 300 mg strength are available. Initially 300 mg given once daily thereafter 75 mg/day.

3. Ticlopidine

It is a prodrug which upon metabolism in liver gets converted into active metabolite. It shows cumulative effect and onset of action is slow (3–5 days). It is available in oral tablets and used as 250 mg twice daily.

Uses

Unstable angina, coronary artery bypass surgery, prophylaxis of myocardial infarction and secondary prevention of stroke.

D. THROMBOLYTIC/FIBRINOLYTIC DRUGS

Q 1. What are thromolytic drugs? Describe any three thrombolytic drugs. OR Write a note on 'thrombolytics/fibrinolytics'.

Thrombolytics

- The agents that are used to break up the thrombi are called thrombolytics.
- They are called fibrinolytics because the breaks fibrin thread in the clot.
- Thrombolytics dissolve both pathological thrombus and fibrin deposits at sites of vascular injury.
- Thrombolytics are used in the treatment of acute myocardial infarction, extensive deep vein thrombosis, major pulmonary embolism and acute arterial occlusion.
- Examples of thrombolytics (fibrinolytics):

  i. Streptokinase   ii. Urokinase   iii. Alteplase

1. Streptokinase

- Streptokinase was discovered in 1933 by Tillett and Garner which was derived from bacterial organisms.
- Streptokinase is a protein produced by β-hemolytic streptococci.

Mechanism of Action

- Streptokinase activates conversion of plasminogen to plasmin (fibrinolysin), fibrinolysin breakdown clots (fibrin).
- Plasmin acts directly on fibrin breaking it down.

Uses

1. In myocardial infarction
2. In thromboembolism
3. In life-threatening deep vein thrombosis
4. In pulmonary embolism
5. In acute arterial thromboembolism
6. In thrombosis of arteries.

Side Effects

- Hypersensitivity
- Surgery
- Parturition
- Trauma
- Heavy vaginal bleeding
- Severe hypertension

2. Urokinase

- Urokinase is a thrombolytic enzyme.
- It is obtained from human urine.
- It is now prepared from cultured human kidney cells.

Mechanism of Action

Urokinase promotes thrombolysis by directly converting plasminogen to plasmin, break down clots.

Uses

It is used in the treatment of:

i. Acute myocardial infarction
ii. Pulmonary embolism
iii. Venous thrombosis

Adverse Effects

- Nausea, vomiting, headache, fever
- Shortness of breath, bronchospasm
- Cyanosis, hypertension
- Skin rash, urticaria
- Itching, flushing
- Anaphylaxis.

Contraindications

- Hypersensitivity
- Severe hypertension
- Pregnancy
- Liver disease
- Cerebral embolism
- Chronic obstructive pulmonary disease (COPD).

3. Alteplase

- Alteplase is tissue plasmogen activator.
- It is obtained or synthesized from human tissue culture, i.e. cultured melanoma cells by DNA technology.
- Alteplase is used to avoid bleeding caused by streptokinase and urokinase.

Mechanism of Action

Alteplase produces fibrin conversion of plasminogen to plasmin, able to bind to fibrin, converts plasminogen in thrombus to plasmin.

Uses

1. In lysis of occlusive coronary artery thrombi associated with acute myocardial infarction.
2. In ischaemic conditions requiring thrombolysis.

Side Effects

- Skin rash, urticaria
- Bradycardia
- Surface bleeding
- Intracranial bleeding

Contraindications

- GIT bleeding
- Hypertension
- Recent trauma
- Pregnancy, lactation.

QUESTIONS: GIVE THE REASONS

Q 1. Why vitamin B_{12} injection is given in pernicious anaemia?

i. Pernicious anaemia is a vitamin B_{12} deficiency due to lack of 'intrinsic factor' of castle secreted by the normal gastric mucosa.
ii. This intrinsic factor is responsible for absorption of dietary vitamin B_{12}.
iii. On oral administration of vitamin B_{12} due to lack of intrinsic factor adequate absorption of vitamin B_{12} will not occur.
iv. On intravenous administration of vitamin B_{12}, there is prompt increase in number of circulating reticulocytes.
v. The bone marrow changes its appearance from megaloblastic to normoblastic, indicating that haemopoiesis is being normalised.
vi. Therefore, vitamin B_{12} injection is given in pernicious anaemia.

Q 2. In overdose of dicoumarol vitamin K is antidote. Why?

i. Vitamin K is useful as a coagulant.
ii. It promotes the synthesis of prothrombin and factors VII, IX and X in the liver.
iii. Dicoumarol is an anticoagulant drug, the overdose of which produces deficiency of vitamin K.
iv. Dicoumarol acts as antimetabolite of vitamin K.
Therefore, in overdose of dicoumarol vitamin K is antidote.

Q 3. Why dextran is given by IV drip?

i. Dextran is a polysaccharide elaborated by microorganism (leuconostoc mesenteroides) seeded in a solution of cane sugar with yeast.
ii. It takes about a week for dextran to be absorbed slowly.
iii. When it is administered, parenterally, remains in bloodstream and increases circulatory fluid volume by exerting an osmotic pressure.
iv. Dextran is a potent antigen when administered in small doses by subcutaneous route.

Objective Questions with Answers in Bold Letters

1. **Anaemia** means decrease in oxygen carrying capacity of blood.
2. The process of formation of RBCs in the red bone marrow is called **erythropoiesis/haemopoiesis**.
3. Megaloblastic anaemia is caused due to deficiency of **vitamin B_{12}**.
4. The drugs with increase the number of RBC or percentage of haemoglobin

in the blood are called **haematinics**.

5. **Desferrioxamine** is an antidote for iron poisoning.
6. **Cyanocobalamin** is also known as antipernicious anaemia agent.
7. **Mitchell** in 1941 isolated folic acid from spinach.
8. The drugs which prevent coagulation/clotting of blood are called **anticoagulants**.
9. Heparin is a **parenteral** anticoagulant.
10. Warfarin and dicoumarol are **oral anticoagulants**.
11. Heparin is a complex **mucopolysaccharide** with a large number of sulphate groups.
12. **Alopecia** is an adverse effect of heparin.
13. Heparin inhibits the activity of **activated factor X**.
14. Haemophilia is a **bleeding disorder**.
15. Oral anticoagulants take about **36–48 hours** for the anticoagulant effect.
16. Oral anticoagulants act by competitively antagonising the actions of **vitamin K**.
17. **Antiplatelet agents** are the drugs which prevent thrombus formation by decreasing platlet aggregation.
18. Antiplatelet agents are also known as **blood thinners**.
19. Aspirin is an **arachidonic acid pathway inhibitor**.
20. Clopidogrel and ticlopidine are the examples of **ADP pathway inhibitors**.
21. The drugs which break down the thrombus are called **thrombolytics**.
22. Streptokinase, urokinase and alteplase are the examples of **fibrinolytics/thrombolytics**.
23. Streptokinase was discovered in 1933 by **Tillett and Garner** which was derived from bacterial organisms.
24. **Alteplase** is a tissue plasminogen activator.
25. Urokinase is a **thrombolytic enzyme**.
26. **Vitamin B_{12} injection** is given in pernicious anaemia.
27. **Dicoumarol** is an anticoagulant drug.
28. Vitamin K is called **coagulation vitamin**.
29. Aspirin is also called **antithrombotic drug**.
30. Clopidogrel inhibits **platelet aggregation**.
31. Coagulants are the drugs which **promote coagulation/clotting**.

Chapter 7

Drugs Acting on Respiratory System

- Bronchodilators
- Expectorants
- Antitussive (anticough) agents
- Mucolytic agents

A. BRONCHODILATORS

Q 1. What is bronchial asthma? Give its treatments.

Bronchial Asthma

Asthma is a chronic disease in which the patient has difficulty in breathing. Bronchial asthma is a clinical syndrome characterised by:

i. Paroxysmal dyspnoea (breathlessness).
ii. Cough due to increased air resistance due to bronchoconstriction.
iii. Narrowing of bronchi is due to bronchospasm, edema of bronchial mucosa and thick sticky mucus in the bronchial lumen.
iv. Hyperreactivity of bronchi which constrict due to allergens.
v. Hypoxemia (decreased arterial O_2 tension).
vi. Hypercapnea (increased arterial CO_2 tension).

The bronchial asthma occurs clinically in three main forms:

1. **Episodic Form:** In this form of asthma, the patient gets acute attacks which are relieved rapidly and completely by bronchodilator drugs with no disability in-between the attacks.
2. **Status Asthmaticus:** In status asthmaticus, an acute attack is severe, persistent and does not respond to adrenaline and aminophylline. It is associated with respiratory insufficiency or failure.
3. **Chronic Form:** In this case, there is a persistent dyspnoea and wheeze of variable severity with acute attacks occurring from time to time.

Treatments

1. Drug treatment: Adrenaline, isoprenaline, terbutaline, corticosteroids.
2. Supporting treatments:
   i. Avoiding respiratory irritants such as tobacco smoking, chemicals.
   ii. Psychological treatment.

iii. Elimination of trigger factors, e.g. allergens.
iv. Ventilation by supply of pure air.
v. Supervision of patient for the physiological parameters like BP, heart rate, pulse, etc.

Q 2. Define and classify bronchodilators with examples. Explain bronchodilators.

Bronchodilators

The drugs which dilate the bronchi and improve the rate of breathing are known as bronchodilators.

Classification

1. Sympathomimetics, e.g. adrenaline, ephedrine, isoprenaline, salbutamol, terbutaline.
2. Phosphodiesterase inhibitors, e.g. theophylline, aminophylline.
3. Anticholinergics, e.g. methyl atropine.

Bronchodilators: The drug therapy in acute attack of asthma involves use of bronchodilators like adrenaline, isoprenaline, salbutamol and aminophylline.

1. Adrenaline Hydrochloride

Adrenaline hydrochloride is potent bronchodilator. It relieves bronchospasm by its action on β-receptors. It is administered subcutaneously in the dose of 0.2–0.5 ml of a 1:1000 aqueous solution. The drug is injected slowly. The relief with adrenaline is accompanied by unpleasant palpitation. Care is to be taken that the tip of needle should not enter into vein. Use of adrenaline in patients with cardiac diseases is dangerous. Administration of adrenaline immediately after inhalation of isoprenaline can cause sudden death. Prolonged use of adrenaline may result in adrenaline resistance.

2. Isoprenaline

Isoprenaline acts similarly as adrenaline and is administered sublingually in the dose of 10–20 mg. It is convenient to take. It acts as rapidly as adrenaline. It has same risk as that of adrenaline, because of its prominent cardiac stimulant action. It can also be given by inhalation route. Isoprenaline largely has been replaced by other sympathomimetic drugs.

3. Salbutamol

Salbutamol is chemically related to isoprenaline. It selectively stimulates β_2-receptors and causes bronchodilation and relaxation of vascular and uterine smooth muscles. It is a poor cardiac stimulant. The selectivity of action makes it a useful agent for treatment of bronchial asthma. It is used as prophylaxis and treatment of asthma, premature labour.

4. Aminophylline and Theophylline

Aminophylline is highly effective in adrenaline resistant patients. It acts directly on smooth muscles.

Aminophylline is used in chronic asthma including nocturnal asthma, acute severe asthma.

Q 3. What is status asthmaticus? Give the signs, symptoms and treatment of status asthmaticus.

Status Asthmaticus

It is a serious medical emergency requiring urgent hospitalisation and vigorous therapy.

Signs and Symptoms

1. Marked dyspnoea
2. Exhaustion
3. Dehydration
4. Tachycardia
5. Respiratory infections
6. Hypoxemia
7. Hypercapnoea

Treatments

1. Hydrocortisone and its derivatives are life-saving drugs in this case. Hydrocortisone 100–200 mg is given parenterally and repeated every one to two hours.
2. Adrenaline and aminophylline are also used.
3. Oxygen is administered in high dosage for the treatment of hypoxemia.
4. Administration of 5% glucose is essential.
5. Isoprenaline aerosol by positive pressure ventilation is applied when all treatments have been failed.
6. The use of antibiotics to overcome associated infections.
7. Rehydration of patient by plenty of fluids orally or by IV infusion.

B. ANTITUSSIVE (ANTICOUGH) AGENTS

Q 1. What is cough? Define and classify antitussive agents.

Pharmacotherapy of Cough

- Cough is a protective reflex which helps to expel irritant matter from respiratory tract.
- Irritation of respiratory tract produces impulses which are carried to cough centre in the medulla oblongata which initiates coughing.

- The act of coughing involves initial deep inspiration followed by forced expiration against temporarily closed glottis.
- When the glottis opens suddenly, the pulmonary air is forced through trachea to expel out foreign material.
- The cough may be productive associated with sputum or dry without much sputum.

Causes

1. Upper respiratory tract infection.
2. Acute lung infectious asthma.
3. Chronic pulmonary diseases, e.g. bronchitis, tuberculosis.
4. Secondary to acute left ventricular failure.

Antitussives (Anticough)

The drugs which are used in the treatment of cough are called antitussives, e.g. noscapine, tincture of opium, heroin, methadone.

Classification

1. Pharyngeal demulscent, e.g. syrups and linctus (codeine linctus).
2. Expectorants, e.g. ammonium chloride, ipecac, ammonium bicarbonate.
3. Central cough suppressants, e.g. noscapine, codeine.

Q 2. Write in brief about 'central cough suppressants'.

Central Cough Suppressants

Central cough suppressants inhibit cough reflex by depressing the cough centre in the medulla. These are mainly useful in the treatment of dry irritant cough. These may be prescribed alone or in combination with expectorants.

1. **Codeine:** Codeine is capable of depressing the cough centre like morphine, due to this reason it is used for this purpose. It can also be used as analgesic. It is relatively safe drug and its adverse effect is constipation.

   Dose: 12 mg codeine phosphate in 4 ml syrup or linctus.
2. **Noscapine:** It is also opium alkaloid belonging to benzyl isoquinoline group. It has smooth muscle relaxant activity and in large doses it acts as bronchodilator. Its antitussive action is equal to that of codeine. It does not produce constipation or narcosis. It is highly effective and probably the safest antitussive.

   All cough suppressants are dangerous in the presence of excessive secretion which may cause mechanical obstruction in respiration. Due to this, these are contraindicated in pleural disease and respiratory failure.

C. EXPECTORANTS

Q 1. What are expectorants? Explain in brief expectorants.

Expectorants

- The drugs which increase the bronchial secretions and help to protect the irritated mucosa are called expectorants.
- Expectorants are the drugs which cause production of demulscent respiratory tract fluid that covers and protects the irritated mucosa.
- These drugs are useful in the treatment of useless cough due to irritation and need liquefaction.
- **Examples of expectorants:** Ammonium chloride, potassium iodide, ammonium bicarbonate, ipecac, guaifenesin.
  1. **Potassium Iodide:** It is used as expectorant to liquefy thick and tenacious sputum. However, iodide-induced goiter and hypothyroidism have been observed. Hence, it is suggested to use alternative drugs when expectorant action is desired.
     Dose: 300 mg with a glassful of water every 4–6 hours.
  2. **Guaifenesin:** White crystalline powder having bitter taste and soluble in water. Studies have shown that guaifenesin used as expectorant relieves dry unproductive cough. It increases respiratory tract secretions. It is an ingredient in a number of expectorant formulations.
     Dose: Usual adult dose is 100–200 mg, every 3–4 hours.
  3. **Ipecac (Ipecacuanha):** The dried rhizome and roots of cephaelis acuminata. The main constituents found in the drug are alkaloids, viz. emetine, cephaeline, psychotrine and ipecamine. It has expectorant, emetic and amoebicidal properties. Ipecac syrup is used as emetic and nauseant expectorant.
     Dose: Emetic dose is 10–30 ml usually 15 ml of ipecac syrup. While expectorant dose is 0.5–2 ml, every six hours.

D. MUCOLYTIC AGENTS

Q 1. Describe mucolytic agents/mucolytics.

Mucolytics

Mucolytics are a class of drugs used to break up and thin mucus, making it easier to clear from the airways.

Categories

a. Expectorants which increase airway water to help with mucus cleaning.
b. Mucoregulators which increase the movement of mucus via cough.
c. Mucokinetics which suppress the mechanisms causing excess mucus secretions.

The important mucolytics used in practice are:

1. Acetylcysteine
2. Bromhexine
3. Ambroxol
4. Carbocisteine
5. Mucinex (guaifenesin)

1. Acetylcysteine

White crystalline powder soluble in water and having acetic odour and sour taste. It reduces the viscosity of pulmonary secretions and facilitate their removal, hence used in bronchopulmonary disorders requiring mucolysis. It is thought that sulfhydryl groups of the drug attack and open up the disulfide bonds in mucus, making it thin.

Uses/Indications

As mucolytic agent for adjunctive therapy of respiratory tract disorders such as chronic obstructive airway disease.

Dosage

Oral tablet/capsule of acetylcysteine 600 mg, once daily. For inhalation of nebulized solution 10% and 20% solutions are available.

Dose: 2–20 ml of 10% solution by inhalation with nebulizer or 1–10 ml of 20% solution by inhalation with nebulizer.

2. Bromhexine

It is a mucolytic agent that breaks up thick and sticky mucus. It is used in combination with dextromethorphan and phenylpropanolamine to treat dry cough associated with cold/flu, allergies or throat irritants. It helps to relieve congestion.

Adverse Effects

Irritation of ear, allergic skin rash, dizziness and headache. It should be used with caution in patients with kidney and liver disorders.

Dosage

It is available in tablets, solutions, syrup and elixir formulations. The usual dose is 8–16 mg, three times in a day.

3. Ambroxol

It is a metabolite of bromhexine. It is used in neonatal respiratory distress syndrome. It breaks up thick viscid mucus and promotes mucus clearance, easing the productive cough. It is one of the active ingredients of cough syrups. It is used in combination with cetirizine, guaifenesin and salbutamol.

Uses

It is effective in relieving cough associated with COPD, emphysema and bronchitis.

Dosage

It is available in tablets, capsules and in syrup formulations. The usual dose is 75 mg once daily.

4. Carbocisteine

It is a mucolytic agent, as it makes the mucus, thin and less sticky. It is used in pulmonary disorders such as COPD and cystic fibrosis. It is a mucoactive drug with free radical scavanging and anti-inflammatory properties. In fact, it is approved for mucolytic properties. The side effects are rare but may be observed in few patients and include allergic skin reactions including anaphylaxis, diarrhoea, nausea, epigastric discomfort and gastrointestinal bleeding.

Dosage

It is available in the form of capsules and liquid orals.

Objective Questions with Answers in Bold Letters

1. Bronchodilators are used in the treatment of **bronchial asthma.**
2. Salbutamol selectively stimulates **β_2-receptors** and causes bronchodilation.
3. **Hydrocortisone** is a drug of choice in status epilepticus.
4. **Adrenaline** is used in bronchial asthma.
5. Syrups and linctus are the examples of **pharyngeal demulscents.**
6. **Noscapine** is an example of central cough suppressant.
7. The drugs which increase bronchial secretions and protect irritated mucosa are called **expectorants.**
8. **Guaifenesin** is an expectorant that relieves dry unproductive cough.
9. Bromhexine is a **mucolytic agent.**
10. **Bronchial asthma** is a paroxysmal dysponea and wheeze described as a result of an increase in respiratory resistance in narrower bronchus.
11. **Cough** is a response that helps to remove irritants from the airway.
12. **Ephedrine** is beneficial for the termination of nocturnal asthma attack in oral doses of 30 mg at bed time.
13. **Ipratropium bromide** is an anticholinergic bronchodilator drug.
14. Nasal decongestants should not produce **nasal irritation.**

Chapter 8

Drugs Acting on Gastrointestinal Tract

- Antiulcer drugs
- Laxatives and purgatives
- Antiemetics
- Antidiarrhoeal drugs

A. ANTIULCER DRUGS

Q 1. What is peptic ulcer? Define and classify antiulcer drugs with examples.

Peptic Ulcer

Peptic ulcer disease refers to painful sores in the mucosal lining of the stomach (gastric ulcer) or the first part of the small intestine (duodenal ulcer).

Causes

- Excessive use of alcohol, tea and coffee.
- Excessive use of certain drugs like corticosteroids, reserpine and indomethacin.

Symptoms

- Heartburn
- Nausea
- Haemorrhage.

Drugs used in Peptic Ulcer

Cimetidine, ranitidine, famotidine, pantoprazole, omeprazole, magnesium hydroxide, aluminium hydroxide.

Antiulcer Drugs

The drugs which are used in the prevention and treatment of peptic ulcer disease are called antiulcer drugs.

Classification

1. **Drugs Reducing Gastric Acid Secretions:**
   i. *Histamine H_2-receptor antagonists:* Cimetidine, ranitidine, famotidine, nizatidine.
   ii. *Proton pump inhibitors (PPI):* Omeprazole, esomeprazole, lansoprazole, rabeprazole, pantoprazole.
   iii. *Ariticholinergics:* Piranzepine, propantheline
   iv. *Prostaglandin analogs:* Misoprostol, enprostil

2. **Antacids, the drugs that neutralize gastric acid:**
   i. *Systemic antacids:* Sodium bicarbonate, sodium citrate.
   ii. *Non-systemic (local) antacids:* Magnesium hydroxide, magnesium trisilicate, aluminium hydroxide gel.
3. **Mucosal protectives:** Sucralfate, CBS (colloidal bismuth subcitrate).
4. **Ulcer healing drugs:** Carbenoxolone sodium.
5. **Antibiotics against *H. pylori*:** Amoxicillin, clarithromycin, metronidazole, tinidazole, tetracycline.

Q 2. Write a note on 'antiulcer drugs' that reduce gastric acid secretion.

Antiulcer Drugs that Reduce Gastric Acid Secretion

1. H_2-receptor Antagonist

Ranitidine: It is a H_2-receptor antagonist which blocks the H_2-receptor of parietal cells.

After ingestion of food in stomach stimulates release of histamine which secretes gastric acid. Ranitidine is a H_2-receptor blocker, so it inhibits the gastric secretion.

Therapeutic uses/Indications

1. In the treatment of gastric and duodenal ulceration.
2. In gastroesophageal reflux.
3. In Zollinger-Ellison syndrome.

Contraindications

- Porphyria
- Pregnancy

2. Proton Pump Inhibitors (PPIs)

These are the group of drugs that act on cell lining of the stomach, reducing the production of acid.

They irreversibly inhibit stomach's H^+/K^+ ATPase proton pump.

Therapeutic uses/Indications

1. In gastric and duodenal ulcers
2. In erosive esophagitis
3. In gastroesophageal reflux disease (GERD)
4. In Zollinger-Ellison syndrome
5. In duodenal ulcer.

Dosage: Lansoprazole 15 mg daily orally

3. Anticholinergics

Cholinergic muscarinic receptor M_1 selective antagonists such as pirenzepine and telenzepine can reduce gastric secretion and hence used in treatment of peptic ulcer.

4. Prostaglandin Analogs

Prostaglandin synthesized by gastric mucosa binds to EP_3 receptors on parietal cells and decreases gastric acid secretion. PGE_2 also prevents gastric injury by cytoprotective effect.

Q 3. Define and classify antacids with examples. Give the qualities of an ideal/good antacid.

Antacids

The drugs which are used to neutralize excessive acidity in the stomach are called antacids.

Classification

A. On the Basis of Site

1. **Oral antacids:** These are the agents having an alkaline reaction which neutralize abnormal acidity in the mouth and are commonly used in dental practice.
2. **Gastric antacids:** These are the agents used to diminish the quantity of hydrochloric acid (HCl) in the stomach and to give relief from peptic ulcer. They act by three mechanisms:
   i. Direct neutralisation, e.g. sodium bicarbonate.
   ii. Buffering of the gastric acid, e.g. sodium citrate, magnesium trisilicate.
   iii. A combination of absorption of H^+ of hydrochloric acid, buffering and partial neutralisation of acid, e.g. hydrated aluminium oxide, anion exhange resins.

B. On the Basis of their Action

1. **Systemic antacids (water soluble)**, e.g. sodium bicarbonate.
2. **Non-systemic antacids (water insoluble)**, e.g. magnesium hydroxide, aluminium hydroxide gel, magnesium trisilicate, calcium carbonate, magnesium oxide.

Properties of an Ideal Antacid

1. It should have a capacity to neutralize excessive acidity.
2. It should have a quick and prolonged action.

3. It should not cause alkalosis.
4. It should be nontoxic, palatable, cheap and easily available.
5. It should not cause constipation or diarrhoea.
6. It should not interfere with digestion and absorption of food.
7. It should not cause evolution of gas.

Q 4. What are the principles of line of treatment of peptic ulcer?

- Peptic ulcer is one of the common diseases of adult male.
- It is caused as a result of digestive action of pepsin and dilute HCl against which the normal stomach and duodenum are protected by their mucus secretions.
- In peptic ulcer, there is an excessive secretion of gastric acid.
- The treatment of peptic ulcer consists of:
  i. Controlling gastric acidity, hypermotility and spasms.
  ii. Promoting ulcer healing.
  iii. Use of antacids, milk or ion exchange resin.
  iv. Withdrawal of stimulants of gastric acid like alcohol, tobacco, etc.
  v. Surgical removal of acid producing gastric mucosa.

Drug Treatments

i. Aluminium hydroxide gel
ii. Magnesium hydroxide
iii. Aluminium trisilicate
iv. Magnesium oxide
v. Ranitidine
vi. Cimetidine
vii. Famotidine.

Q 5. Write a note on 'systemic and non-systemic antacids'.

Systemic and Non-systemic Antacids

A. **Systemic antacids:** Systemic antacids directly neutralise the hydrochloric acid (HCl) of gastric juice. They are highly soluble, readily absorbable and capable of altering the pH of blood towards alkalinity on prolonged use.

Sodium Bicarbonate ($NaHCO_3$)

It provides prompt relief from the symptoms of hyperacidity by direct neutralization.

$$NaHCO_3 + HCl \rightarrow NaCl + H_2O + CO_2 \uparrow$$

Due to neutralisation of HCl in the stomach, $NaHCO_3$ secreted along with alkaline juices in the intestine remains unneutralised and gets absorbed as such. In addition to this, large amount of $NaHCO_3$ when administered also gets absorbed and ultimately causing disturbance of acid–base balance of body. Interaction of $NaHCO_3$ and HCl causes release of CO_2; which may cause distension of stomach and sometimes perforation of peptic ulcer. CO_2 released also stimulates the secretion of gastric juice which causes rebound acidity. $NaHCO_3$ also dissolves the mucous plug of gastric glands thus causing a free flow of gastric juice. The action of $NaHCO_3$ is shortlived followed by aggravation of symptoms.

B. **Non-systemic antacids:** These are insoluble, non-absorbable and not capable of altering the pH of blood. The action of non-systemic antacids is confined locally and are therefore, preferred in clinical practice, e.g. magnesium trisilicate, aluminium hydroxide.

1. **Magnesium trisilicate:** The action is confined locally in the stomach. The drug acts by direct neutralisation as well as by buffering and adsorption mechanism. On account of reaction with HCl it forms $MgCl_2$ and SiO_2. The latter has gelatinous consistency and forms a protective covering over the ulcers. $MgCl_2$ is passed on to the intestine where it reacts with $NaHCO_3$ of the alkaline juice forming NaCl which is absorbed as normally. The chemical reactions taking place in the stomach and intestine are as follows;

$$2\,(MgO)\,3\,(SiO_2) + 4HCl + nH_2O \rightarrow 2\,MgCl_2 + 3SiO_2 + (n+2)\,H_2O$$

Intestine

$$2\,NaHCO_3 + MgCl_2 \rightarrow MgCO_3 + 2\,NaCl + CO_2\uparrow + H_2O$$

Action is confined to stomach. There is no liberation of CO_2 in the stomach. The drug does not affect absorption of other substances in the stomach. The onset of action is rapid and sustained. The drug does not affect the pH of blood. Mg^{2+} exerts high osmotic pressure in the gut causing retention of water resulting in diarrhoea.

2. **Aluminium hydroxide $Al(OH)_3$:** It is available both as a suspension in water as well as dry powder. It resembles magnesium trisilicate in its action. It neutralises acidity by direct neutralisation, buffering and adsorption. Reaction with HCl in the stomach leads to formation of $AlCl_3$ which reacts with $NaHCO_3$ in intestine to form $Al(OH)_3$ and NaCl. NaCl is reabsorbed while $Al(OH)_3$ is excreted in faeces.

   Stomach: $Al(OH)_3 + 3\,HCl \rightarrow AlCl_3 + 3\,H_2O$

   Intestine: $3\,NaHCO_3 + AlCl_3 \rightarrow Al(OH)_3 + 3\,NaCl + 3CO_2\uparrow$

Action is confined to stomach. There is no liberation of CO_2 in stomach. The drug does not cause diarrhoea. It has a sustained action. On account of its astringent action it diminishes the gut of gastric juice secreted. It does not affect pH of blood. The drug may cause constipation. It may also prevent absorption of vitamins A and B, proteins, phosphates and tetracyclins.

B. ANTIEMETICS

Q 1. What is emesis? Define and classify antiemetics with examples.

Emesis (vomiting)

Emesis is the forceful expulsion of the contents of the stomach through the mouth and sometimes the nose.

Nausea: It is a feeling of emesis.

Causes

1. Gastritis (inflammation of the gastric wall, usually by viruses)
2. Food poisoning
3. Bowel obstruction
4. Overeating
5. Food allergies
6. Gastroenteritis
7. Motion sickness
8. Stimulation of CTZ
9. Local irritation in GIT
10. Vestibular stimulation
11. Psychological

Antiemetics

The drugs which prevent vomiting are called antiemetics.

Classification

1. 5-HT_3 receptor antagonist, e.g. ondansetron, granisetron.
2. Dopamine D_2 receptor antagonist, e.g. metoclopramide, promethazine.
3. H_1 antihistaminics, e.g. cyclizine, meclozine.
4. Muscarinic receptor antagonists (anticholinergics), e.g. hyoscine, scopolamine.
5. Cannabinoids
6. Steroids.

Q 2. Describe in brief 'centrally acting dopamine receptor antagonists'.

Centrally acting dopamine receptor antagonists, e.g. metoclopramide, promethazine, chlorpromazine.

1. Metoclopramide

The antiemetic action of metoclopramide is due to its D_2 receptor antagonist activity in the CTZ.

Therapeutic uses/Indications

1. To prevent vomiting in GI disorders
2. Chemotherapy-induced emesis
3. Pre- and post-operative vomiting
4. Nausea and vomiting in migraine
5. In gastroesophageal reflux

Contraindications

- GI obstructions
- Haemorrhage or perforation
- Convulsive disorders

Dosage

1. Metoclopramide tablet : 10 mg, twice daily
2. Metoclopramide injection : 3 mg/kg by IV every 2 hours.

2. Promethazine

In addition to D_2 dopaminergic receptor blockade, it has histamine H_1 and muscarinic receptor blocking properties.

Therapeutic uses/Indications

1. To treat motion sickness.
2. In allergic conditions of respiratory tract, e.g. sneezing.
3. In conditions like snake bite, urticaria.
4. To treat insomnia.
5. As a preanaesthetic medication.
6. As antiemetic.
7. In various cough preparations.

Adverse Effects

Nausea, vomiting, labyrinth disorders.

Contraindications: Porphyria.

Dosage: Promethazine HCl tablet 10 mg orally

Brand name: Avomin

Q 3. What are emetics and antiemetics? Give the examples and uses of emetics and antiemetics.

Emetics

The drugs which induce vomiting are called emetics.

Emesis: It is the process of vomiting. It can be caused due to:

- i. Stimulation of CTZ
  ii. Local irritation in GIT
  iii. Vestibular stimulation
  iv. Psychological

Drugs: Apomorphine, ipecac, mustard, sodium chloride solution.

Uses

i. In poisoning cases for gastric lavage
ii. As expectorants.

Antiemetics

The drugs which prevent vomiting are called antiemetics, e.g. metoclopramide, promethazine, domperidone.

Uses

i. In vomiting due to poisoning
ii. Preanaesthetic medication
iii. To prevent vomiting of pregnancy
iv. In motion sickness.

C. LAXATIVES AND PURGATIVES

Q 1. What is constipation? Name the drugs used in the treatment of constipation.

Constipation

Constipation is a condition in which defaecation is delayed and hard stools are formed due to reabsorption of large amount of water from intestinal contents.

Causes/Reasons

1. Obstruction in bowel
2. Due to hypothyroidism
3. Due to certain drugs such as atropine, morphine, calcium channel blockers.

Drugs used in the Treatment

1. Senna, castor oil
2. Bisacodyl
3. Magnesium sulphate
4. Sodium potassium tartrate
5. Aloe
6. Phenolphthalein.

Q 2. Define purgatives and laxatives. Classify them with suitable examples.

Purgatives: The drugs which promote defaecation are called purgatives.

Laxatives: Laxatives are mild purgatives.

Cathartics: Cathartics are strong purgatives.

- Purgatives are also known as laxatives or aperients.
- These drugs induce bowel movement or loosen the stools.
- Purgatives and laxatives are mainly used in the treatment of constipation.
- The terms purgatives, laxatives and cathartics are used synonymously.

Classification

a. ***Irritant purgatives:***
   - i. Anthracene group, e.g. rhubarb, senna, aloe.
   - ii. Drastic purgatives, e.g. croton oil, podophyllum.
   - iii. Mild purgatives, e.g. castor oil, phenolphthalein, bisacodyl.

b. ***Bulk purgatives:***
   - i. Saline purgatives (osmotic purgatives), e.g. magnesium sulphate, sodium potassium tartrate, potassium phosphate.
   - ii. Methyl cellulose, sodium carboxymethyl cellulose, plantago, agar-agar.

c. ***Lubricant purgatives***, e.g. mineral oil (liquid paraffin), dioctyl sodium sulphosuccinate.

Q 3. Write a note on 'irritant/stimulant purgatives (laxatives)'.

Irritant/Stimulant Purgatives

These are the substances that are themselves irritant or contain an irritant substance to produce purgation. They are the strongest and most abused laxative products that act by irritating the GI mucosa and pulling water into the bowel lumen, e.g. senna, castor oil, rhubarb, phenolphthalein, bisacodyl.

a. **Phenolphthalein:** It acts mainly on colon though the small intestine may also be stimulated. The onset of action is about 6–8 hours. The exact mechanism of action is not known. A small portion may be absorbed and excreted in bile which may prolong its action. The drug is relatively nontoxic. Excessive amounts may cause severe diarrhoea resulting in fluid imbalance.

b. **Bisacodyl (Dulcolax):** It has structural similarity to phenolphthalein and effective orally as well as rectally. It is not absorbed from digestive tract and no systemic effects have been reported. Precise mechanism of action is not known. But the stimulant action on colon appears to be resultant of a direct contact with wall of colon. The usual oral dose is 10–15 mg for adults and 5–10 mg for children.

c. **Castor oil:** Castor oil is a fixed oil obtained from the seeds of *Ricinus communis*. Chemically, it is triglyceride of ricinoleic acid. When taken orally it is hydrolysed by intestinal lipase to glycerol and ricinoleic acid. The latter stimulates the peristaltic movement of small intestine. Full dose of castor oil produces purgation within 2–6 hours. Larger dose does not produce excessive purgation because most of the excess remains unhydrolysed which is absorbed and metabolised like other fatty acids. The castor oil is relatively a safe cathartic. Dose is 5–15 ml early in the morning before morning breakfast.

Q 4. Write a note on 'saline purgative/osmotic purgative'.

Saline Purgatives

- These drugs act by maintaining a volume of fluid in the bowel by osmosis.
- These drugs increase the osmotic pressure by secreting additional fluid in the intestinal tract resulting in increase in bulk and stimulate the peristalsis of GIT, hence they are used in constipation.
- These are the salts which are poorly or incompletely absorbed from the gut. Commonly used salts are a number of magnesium salts, various sulphates and tartrates. The intensity of action and onset of action vary with the individual salt. When given in full doses the action occurs within 3–6 hours. When large amount of these salts is given they exert high osmotic pressure and retain large amount of water in the gut lumen which exerts mechanical stimulus to increase the intestinal peristalsis. The efficacy of saline purgative depends on the osmotic pressure exerted by unabsorbed fraction in the intestinal lumen. A small fraction of ingested salt may be absorbed, but is readily excreted through the kidney. However, in case of kidney dysfunction, it may be retained and may cause magnesium intoxication. Thus, in patients suffering from severe kidney dysfunction, magnesium salts should be avoided as purgatives. On the other hand, in cases of congestive cardiac failure, sodium salts should be avoided.

Examples

i. Magnesium sulphate : 5–15 gm before breakfast.
ii. Magnesium carbonate : 2–4 gm as required.
iii. Magnesium hydroxide : 2–4 gm as required.

Therapeutic uses

1. In constipation.
2. For easy evacuation in patients suffering from painful haemorrhoids or other rectal disorders.
3. To remove radiopaque solid prior to X-ray analysis.
4. To avoid rise in blood pressure during evacuation of bowel.

Q 5. Write in brief about lubricant/emollient purgatives.

Lubricant/Emollient Purgatives

These are the drugs that lubricate the intestine and soften the stool by retarding colonic absorption of fecal water. These are also knwon as fecal softness/stool softners. Examples: Liquid paraffin, mineral oil, dioctyl sodium sulphosuccinate.

1. Liquid Paraffin

- It consists of petrolatum hydrocarbon. Therefore, it is called mineral oil.
- It helps to lubricate and supress the faeces in the intestine.
- It acts by two mechanisms:
  i. Causing lubrication of hard stool by coating.
  ii. Increasing bulk of the intestinal contents as it reduces water absorption.

Therapeutic uses/Indications

1. In the treatment of anal fissure
2. In the treatment of haemorrhoids.

2. Dioctyl Sodium Sulphosuccinate

- It is an anionic surface active agent which has been used in pharmaceutical industry as an emulgent and as a wetting or dispersing agent for external application.
- It was introduced in 1955 with the claim that it promotes formation of soft stool without stimulation of peristalsis.
- It is used in the dose of 30–100 mg daily.

Q 6. Define purgatives/laxatives. Give the indications or therapeutic uses of purgatives and laxatives.

Purgatives

The drugs which promote defaecation are called purgatives.

Indications/Therapeutic uses

1. In treatment of constipation.
2. In food or drug poisoning saline purgatives are used.
3. During anthelmintic therapy, purgatives are given.
4. Used before preoperative abdominal surgery and X-ray examination.
5. In patients with anal fissures, pile and in pregnant women in order to avoid excessive straining during defaecation, the purgatives are given.
6. To accelerate elimination of potentially toxic substances from the GIT.

D. ANTIDIARRHOEAL DRUGS

Q 1. What is diarrhoea? Give its treatments. Define antidiarrhoeal drugs and classify them with examples. OR Write a note on 'antidiarrhoeal drugs'.

Diarrhoea

Diarrhoea is condition characterized by an abnormally frequent discharge of watery stools from the bowel.

Causes

1. The primary cause of diarrhoea is high intestinal motility
2. Infection by bacteria
3. Allergy to certain foods
4. Diseases of the intestine
5. Radiation therapy
6. Hyperthyroidism
7. Medications.

Symptoms

1. Abdominal bloating or cramps
2. Thin or loose stools
3. Watery stools
4. Loss of appetite
5. Fatigue

Treatments

a. **Specific treatment:** The specific cause of diarrhoea can be treated by using specific antibacterial, anthelmintic and antiprotozoal agents.
b. **Symptomatic and supportive therapy:**
   - Use of antidiarrhoeal agents
   - Correction of dehydration and electrolyte disturbances
   - Administration of intravenous fluids
   - Oral rehydration therapy (ORT).

Antidiarrhoeal Drugs

The drugs which are used in the treatment of diarrhoea are called antidiarrhoeal drugs.

Classification/Types

1. Gastrointestinal protectives and adsorbents, e.g. pectin, activated charcoal, light kaolin, bismuth subsalicylate.
2. Drugs affecting gastrointestinal motility, e.g. opioid derivatives (codeine), atropine.
3. Miscellaneous, e.g. loperamide.

1. Gastrointestinal Protectives and Adsorbents

These compounds are used to adsorb harmful substances such as gases, germs and poisons. Some of them also work as astringent, while others prevent irritants from the gastrointestinal membrane by covering it.

a. **Pectin:** When ingested it passes into the intestinal tract where it acts by mechanical coating.

b. **Activated wood charcoal:** Flatulence, dyspepsia and other diarrhoea kinds are commonly employed in treatment. It is also good to treat alkaloid poisoning as a matter of urgency, such as morphine and strychnine. It is commonly given orally at 4–8 gm dose or as a universal antidote component.

c. **Light kaolin:** It acts as an adsorbent of bacteria and bacterial toxins. A mixture containing 20% kaolin with 1% pectin is used in the dose of 30 ml.

2. Drugs Affecting Gastrointestinal Motility

The opiates are strong and reliable inhibitors of bowel propulsion. A dose of 30–60 mg of codeine is used to control GIT motility. In order to treat the diarrhoea accompanied colic, especially atropine, belladonna alkaloids are useful.

Objective Questions with Answers in Bold Letters

1. Ranitidine and cimetidine are the **H_2-receptor antagonists.**
2. PPIs means **proton pump inhibitors.**
3. The drugs which neutralizes excessive acidity in the stomach are called **antacids.**
4. **Magnesium trisilicate** is non-systemic antacid.
5. Emesis is a **process of vomiting.**
6. The drugs which prevent vomiting are called **antiemetics.**
7. The agents which induce vomiting are called **emetics.**
8. Ondansetron is a **5-HT_3 receptor antagonist.**
9. Sodium bicarbonate is a **systemic antacid.**
10. Metoclopramide is an **antiemetic drug.**
11. Promethazine is a drug of choice in **motion sickness.**
12. Avomin is a popular brand name of **promethazine.**
13. **Constipation** is a condition where defaecation is delayed.
14. Bisacodyl is a **purgative drug.**
15. The drugs which promote defaecation are called **purgatives.**
16. **Castor oil** is an irritant/stimulant purgative.
17. Liquid paraffin is an **emollient purgative.**
18. Magnesium sulphate is a **saline/osmetic** purgative.
19. A popular brand name of bisacodyl is **Dulcolax.**
20. **Purgatives** are used in the treatment of constipation.

Chapter 9

Drugs Acting on Kidney

• Diuretics • Antidiuretics

A. DIURETICS

Q 1. Define and classify diuretics giving suitable examples. Give the indications/uses of diuretics.

Diuretics

The drugs which increase the formation and excretion of urine are called diuretics.

Classification

1. **Weak diuretics:**
   a. Osmotic diuretics
      i. Electrolytes, e.g. sodium and potassium salts
      ii. Non-electrolytes, e.g. mannitol
   b. Acidifying salts, e.g. ammonium chloride
   c. Xanthine derivatives, e.g. aminophylline
   d. Carbonic anhydrase inhibitors, e.g. acetazolamide
2. **Moderately potent diuretics,** e.g. benzothiadiazine.
3. **Very potent diuretics,** e.g. parenteral organic mercurials (mercaptomerin, mersalyl), frusemide, ethacrynic acid.
4. **Potassium sparing diuretics,** e.g. triameterene, amiloride, spironolactone.

Indications of Diuretic Therapy (Therapeutic/Clinical uses)

Diuretics are indicated in the following conditions:

1. In edema
2. In hypertension
3. In congestive heart failure
4. In glaucoma
5. In diabetes insipidus
6. In salicylate and barbiturate poisoning

Q 2. Write a note on "osmotic diuretics".

Osmotic Diuretics

a. ***Electrolytes:*** Capacity of tubules to reabsorb osmotically active substances is limited. If in plasma, one of such solute is increased then its concentration in glomerular filtrate also increases. Thus, increase in concentration of solute in the tubular fluid opposes the reabsorption of water by osmotic activity and acts as an osmotic diuretic. Thus, increase in excretion of such solute increases excretion of water. Thus, osmotic diuretic should not get metabolised in the body and should not get reabsorbed by renal tubules.

1. **Sodium chloride (NaCl):** Excess of NaCl causes osmotic diuresis. Intravenous administration of hypertonic NaCl solution raises solute concentration of extracellular fluid and of glomerular filtrate leading to diuresis. Sodium salts are however weak in action as Na^+ is reabsorbed. In case of oedema where diuretics are indicated there is already excess Na^+ in body and sodium salts aggravate the condition. $NaHCO_3$ is sometimes used to produce alkaline urine, e.g. in urinary tract infections and in sulphonamide administration.
2. **Potassium salts:** These are more effective than sodium salts. Potassium citrate is commonly used to produce alkaline urine. Administration of potassium salts in presence of renal insufficiency causes hyperkalemia.

b. *Non-electrolytes*

Mannitol

Mannitol is a sugar. When hypertonic solution of mannitol is injected; draws water from the cells and extracellular spaces into the vessels. Plasma volume is increased enhancing renal blood flow and diuresis occurs by increase in osmotic pressure of the glomerular filtrate so that tubular reabsorption of water is diminished. It is used as diuretic to treat oliguric condition of acute renal failure. It is also used to reduce intraocular pressure and to treat cerebral edema.

Contraindications

Pulmonary edema, intracranial bleeding, severe cogestive heart failure, severe dehydration and renal failure.

Dosage

Solution for infusion in 10% and 20% strength is available for raised intracranial and intraocular pressure: By IV infusion of 20% solution infused over 30–60 minutes.

Q 3. Write a note on "acetazolamide as a self-limiting diuretic."

Or

Write a note on carbonic anhydrase inhibitors.

Carbonic Anhydrase Inhibitors

Acetazolamide: It acts by inhibiting the enzyme carbonic anhydrase.

Pharmacological Actions

Kidney and electrolytes: Carbonic anhydrase is present in renal cortex. It catalyses the reaction.

$$CO_2 + H_2O \xrightleftharpoons{\text{Carbonic anhydrase}} H_2CO_2$$

The H_2CO_3 that has generated, dissociates into H^+ and HCO_3^-. This H^+ is made available for Na to swap. As a result, the enzyme is critical for sodium reabsorption in the tubules.

Acetazolamide inhibits this enzyme through a noncompetitive method, preventing H^+ from being exchanged with Na. As a result, the enzyme is critical for sodium reabsorption in the tubules.

Acetazolamide inhibits this enzyme through a noncompetitive method, preventing H^+ from being exchanged for Na^+. As a result, Na^+ is expelled together with water. The H^+ ion reacts with HCO_3 from the glomerular filtrate to produce H_2CO_3, which is then transformed to water and carbon dioxide. The carbon dioxide that has been produced is absorbed. As a result of the absence of H^+, a considerable amount of HCO_3 is expelled, and the urine turns alkaline. Because there are not enough H^+ ions, Na^+ is exchanged for K^+, resulting in K^+ loss. As a result, the acetazolamide produces a loss of Na^+, HCO_3, and K^+. As a result, the extracellular fluid base decreases, resulting in metabolic acidosis. This results in loss of diuretic activity. Hence, acetazolamide is self-limiting diuretics.

Q 4. Write a note on "moderately potent diuretics."

Or

Write a note on benzothiadiazine/thiazide diuretics.

Benzothiadiazine/Thiazide Diuretics

Pharmacological Action/Mechanism of Action

Kidney: These drugs prevent reabsorption of Na^+ and Cl^-. They are believed to act mainly on the site proximal to Na^+ and K^+ exchange region in the distal tubules; the glomerular filtration rate is not affected. Initially, the drug causes decrease in Na^+ reabsorption in the distal tubules and a gradual reduction in extracellular fluid volume. When extracellular fluid volume falls to below normal, the reabsorption of Na^+ from proximal tubule is stimulated. The amount of Na^+ delivered to distal tubule is decreased. This causes decrease in diuretic activity and resistance. Because of strong inhibitory action on Na^+ reabsorption a large amount of Na^+ is made available to distal segment, where exchange of K^+ with Na^+ takes place. This results into increased loss of K^+ ions.

Adverse Effects

1. Hypokalemia
2. Hyponatremia
3. Hypochloremic alkalosis
4. Hyperglycemia

Contraindications

1. In severe renal and hepatic impairment
2. In hyponatremia
3. In refractory hypokalemia
4. In Addison's disease

Uses/Indications

1. It is used in sodium retention edema
2. In diabetes insipidus
3. In hypertension
4. In heart failure

Dosage

1. Chlorthiazide tablet : 500–1000 mg daily **(Brand name:** Diuril)
2. Hydrochlorthiazide tablet : 25–200 mg daily
3. Hydroflumethiazide tablet : 25–200 mg daily

Q 5. Write a note on "parenteral oganic mercurial compounds as a diuretic".

Parenteral organic mercurial compounds: Organic mercurial compounds given parenterally are effective diuretics.

Pharmacological Actions/Mechanism of Action

a. ***Kidney:*** Mercurials act directly at various sites in the nephron. They inhibit the intracellular enzyme and thus depresses the reabsorption of Na^+ and Cl^- causing diuresis. Precise mechanism of action is not known. But it is supposed that internal release of divalent mercury ion is responsible for diuretic property. The mercurial ion has affinity for sulphydryl group. It reacts with sulphydryl group of enzymes responsible for tubular reabsorption of Na^+. As sulphydryl group from enzymes is made inactive the reabsorption of Na^+ decreases causing diuresis. The effect of full dose of mercurial diuresis can be enhanced further by thiazides or aminophylline. Mercurials cause K^+ loss as that of thiazides.

b. ***Other action:*** Mercury is toxic ion and if accumulated in the body is capable of producing mercurial poisoning. These are administered intramuscularly and should never be given intravenously as they may precipitate severe cardiac toxicity. These are rapidly excreted by kidney and the excretion is almost complete by 24 hours.

Adverse Effects

1. Sudden ventricular fibrillation
2. Collapse and death
3. Renal and hepatic damage
4. Hypochloremic alkalosis

Therapeutic uses

1. In the treatment of edema due to nephrosis 2. In congestive heart failure

Dosage

1. Mersalyl injection IP : 0.5–2 ml by IM
2. Mercaptomerin sodium injection : 1 ml by SC or IM once or thrice daily.

Q 6. Write a ntoe on "loop diuretics"/"high ceiling diuretics".

Or

Describe frusemide and ethacrynic acid as a diuretics.

Loop Diuretics

1. ***Frusemide:*** It is a potent oral non-mercurial diuretic.

Pharmacological Action/Mechanism of Action

Kidney and electrolytes: On oral administration the intense diuretic action starts within an hour and is completed in 4–6 hours. It produces more chloride loss than Na^+ loss. The frusemide acts along the entire nephron including the loop of Henle with the exception only of distal site where Na^+ is exchanged for K^+ and H^+. Hence, unlike thiazides the urinary excretion of Na^+ continues even when patient's extracellular fluid volume has been severely depleted. In therapeutic doses, it has little effect on carbonic anhydrase. It causes increased excretion of phosphates. Drug enhances K^+ excretion and causes little change in urinary pH and its diuretic response is not limited by the state of electrolyte, or acid–base balance of the body. The excessive loss of chloride may lead to hypochloremic alkalosis. The K^+ loss may cause hypokalemia.

Adverse Effects

1. Disturbance in electrolyte and water balance of body
2. Weakness, fatigue
3. Hypotension
4. Cardiac arrest
5. Hepatic coma
6. Skin rash, nausea, vomiting, diarrhoea

Therapeutic uses/Indications

1. It is used as diuretic
2. To treat edema associated with CHF; cirrhosis of liver
3. Used for management of hypertension
4. To treat renal disease

Contraindications

- Renal failure with anuria
- Liver cirrhosis

Dosage

Frusemide tablet : 20–80 mg orally.

Brand name: Lasix.

2. *Ethacrynic acid*

- It is very patent oral diuretic.
- When given orally the maximum diuresis occurs within 2–3 hours while on IM administration the effect starts within few minutes.

Adverse Effects

1. Potassium depletion
2. Hypochloremic alkalosis

Therapeutic uses

1. As a diuretic 2. To treat edema 3. In the management of hypertension

Dosage

Ethacrynic acid tablet : 50–100 mg daily.

Q 7. Write a note on "potassium sparing diuretics".

Potassium Sparing Diuretics

These drugs spare the potassium in the body and avoids hypokalemia condition. Hence, called potassium sparing diuretics.

For example: Spironolactone, triamterene, amiloride.

1. Spironolactone

- Spironolactone is an aldosterone antagonist
- It acts by competitive antagonism of aldosterone
- It prevents secretion of potassium and decreasing sodium reabsorption

Therapeutic uses/Indications

1. In hypertension
2. In CHF
3. In refractory edema
4. In nephrotic syndrome
5. Hepatic cirrhosis with edema

Adverse Effects

- Hyperkalemia
- Hyponatremia
- Hyperchloremic acidosis
- Dehydration
- Menstrual irregularities
- Arrhythmias

Contraindications

- In pregnancy
- Breastfeeding
- Hyperkalemia
- Severe renal impairment
- Addison's disease

Dosage

Spironolactone tablet : 100–200 mg daily.

B. ANTIDIURETICS

Q 1. What are antidiuretics? Explain in brief ADH.

Or

Write a note on antidiuretics.

Antidiuretics

The drugs which reduce urine volume are called antidiuretics.

- These drugs are useful in diabetes insipidus.
- *Examples:* ADH (vasopressin), desmopressin, lypressin, oxytocin, chlorpropamide, carbamazepine.

Therapeutic uses/Indications

1. In prevention of postoperative abdominal distension.
2. In abdominal roentgenography.
3. In diabetes insipidus.
4. Desmopressin is used to treat central cranial diabetes insipidus.
5. Desmopressin is used to control bed wetting.

Antidiuretic Hormone (ADH)

- It is released by the posterior lobe of pituitary gland along with oxytocin.
- It has a vasopressor effect so it is called vasopressin.
- The degree of dehydration and circulating blood volume influence the secretion of ADH.

Mechanism of Action

Antidiuretic hormone acts by increasing reabsorption of water in the distal tubules and in the loop of Henle, due to which the amount of water in the urine is decreased. It does not effect the excretion of electrolytes. Antidiuretic hormone is used in the treatment of patients suffering from diabetes insipidus.

Pharmacological Actions

1. ***Action on kidneys:*** Due to the effect of antidiuretic hormone, the distal tubules and collecting duct of nephron become permeable to water which leads to reduction of total volume of urine. The absence of antidiuretic hormone causes the disease diabetes insipidus.
2. ***Action on cardiovascular system:*** In large doses ADH raises blood pressure due to direct stimulation of vascular smooth muscles. Due to direct

depressant effect of antidiuretic hormone, myocardium, blood pressure falls due to narrowing of coronary blood vessels.

3. ***Action on smooth muscles:*** Antidiuretic hormone in large doses stimulates smooth muscles of gastrointestinal tract cause increase in peristalsis. ADH should not be administered orally as it is destroyed by trypsin. It is administered by parenteral route.

Therapeutic uses

1. To treat diabetes insipidus
2. Used in emergency condition to raise blood pressure

Adverse Effects

- Numbness or tingling
- Dizziness
- Stomach pain, nausea, vomiting
- Sweating

Contraindications

- Hypersensitivity
- Vascular disease
- Chronic nephritis

Q 2. Give the dose, route and brand name of following diuretics.

Drug	*Brand name*	*Dose*	*Route*
1. Acetazolamide	Diamox	250–500 mg daily	Oral
2. Frusemide	Lasix	20–80 mg daily	Oral
3. Spironolactone	Aldactone	25–100 mg daily	Oral
4. Chlorthiazide	Diuril	250–1000 mg daily	Oral
5. Mannitol	Osmitrol	50–100 gm (15–20% solution)	IV
6. Triamterene	Dyrenium	100–200 mg daily	Oral

QUESTIONS: GIVE THE REASONS

Q 1. Why water is called physiological diuretic (natural diuretic)?

i. ADH (antidiuretic hormone) is secreted by posterior lobe of pituitary gland.
ii. ADH increases the permeability of distal convoluted tubule and causes more reabsorption of water.
iii. When excess water is taken (excess fluid intake), it causes decrease in the osmotic pressure of blood.
iv. This inhibits the ADH secretion and results into decreased reabsorption of water causing diuresis.

Hence, water is called physiological diuretic/natural diuretic.

Q 2. Why diuretics are given along with antihypertensive drug?

i. One of the causes of hypertension is presence of excess plasma sodium and calcium level.
ii. To eliminate these in the form of salts, diuretics are used.

iii. Diuretics inhibit reabsorption of sodium and its equivalent osmotic amount of water.
iv. This causes decrease in plasma fluid which decreases blood pressure.
v. Diuretics also cause vasodilation and decrease blood pressure. Therefore, diuretics are given along with antihypertensive drugs.

Q 3. Why acetazolamide is self-limiting diuretic?

i. The enzyme carbonic anhydrase is present in renal cortex. It catalyses following reaction:

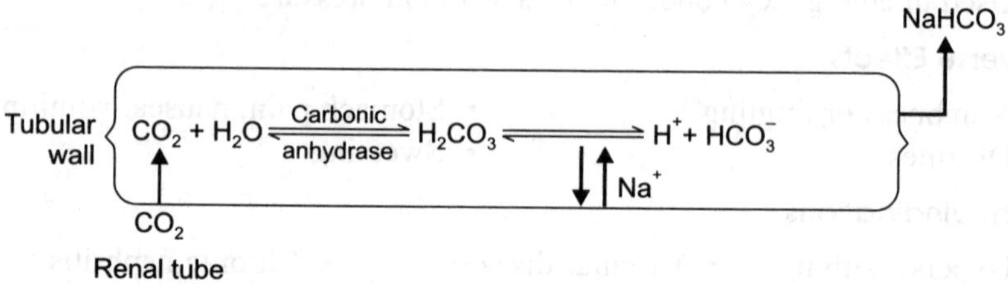

ii. The carbonic acid thus formed in the wall of renal tubule dissociates to give H^+ and HCO_3^-. The H^+ ion formed is secreted in the renal tubule, in the exchange of which Na^+ is reabsorbed.
iii. Acetazolamide inhibits the enzyme by noncompetitive mechanism, so that H^+ is not made available for exchange with Na^+. Hence, Na^+ along with water is excreted.
iv. H^+ ion combines with HCO_3^- provided by glomerular filtrate to form H_2CO_3 which dissociates to form water and carbon dioxide. The carbon dioxide formed is absorbed.
v. Thus, in acetazolamide therapy, due to lack of H^+ and HCO_3^-; is excreted in large amount and the urine becomes alkaline.
vi. Since, there is lack of H^+ ions, Na^+ is exchanged with K^+ which causes loss of potassium.
vii. The acetazolamide thus causes loss of Na^+, HCO_3^-; and K^+.
viii. Thus, there is decrease in extracellular fluid base which causes metabolic acidosis.
ix. This results in loss of diuretic activity. Hence, acetazolamide is self-limiting diuretic.

Q 4. Why potassium salt is given along with thiazide diuretics?

i. Thiazide diuretics prevent reabsorption of Na^+ and Cl^- from proximal convoluted tubule of nephron.
ii. Because of strong inhibitory action on Na^+ reabsorption, large amount of Na^+ is made available to distal segment of the nephron, where exchange of K^+ with Na^+ takes place.

iii. This causes increase in loss of K^+ ions.

iv. Thus, prolonged use of thiazides causes hypokalemia.

v. To overcome this potassium loss, potassium salt is given along with thiazides.

Q 5. Why ammonium chloride is given with organomercurials?

i. Mercurial depresses the active sodium reabsorption in the proximal tubule.

ii. Mercurial causes net loss of sodium, chloride, water and potassium.

iii. This results in fall of chloride and rise of bicarbonate in the plasma called hypochloremic alkalosis.

iv. Ammonium chloride results into acidosis and high concentration of chloride in glomercular filtrate.

v. Hence, ammonium chloride is given as an adjunct to mercurials to overcome the hypochloremic alkalosis.

Q 6. Why toxicity of digitalis is increased by chlorthiazide?

i. Chlorthiazide is a diuretic drug.

ii. Thiazides depress sodium transport in the cortical diluting segment of nephron just proximal to the point of Na–K exchange.

iii. Thiazides also increase potassium excretion to a considerable extent.

iv. In the treatment of congestive cardiac failure with digitalis, there is already excess potassium loss (due to excess sodium retention causing edema), i.e. hypokalemia.

v. Hence, if chlorthiazide diuretics are administered in patients on digitalis therapy then these increase the toxicity of digitalis.

Objective Questions with Answers in Bold Letters

1. **Diuretics** are the drugs which speedup and increase the volume of urine produced.
2. Acetazolamide is a **carbonic anhydrase inhibitor**.
3. Mannitol is a **weak diuretic.**
4. Spironolactone is a **potassium sparing diuretic**.
5. **Acetazolamide** is a self-limiting diuretic.
6. Frusemide and ethacrynic acid are **loop diuretics**.
7. **Lasix** is a popular brand name of frusemide.
8. The drugs which reduce urine volume are called **antidiuretic drugs**.
9. ADH means **antidiuretic hormone** and also called vasopressin.
10. **Antidiuretic drugs** are used in diabetes insipidus.

11. ADH is released by **posterior lobe** of pituitary gland.
12. **Diuretics** are used in the treatment of hypertension and edema.
13. Toxicity of digitalis is increased by **chlorthiazide**.
14. Diuretics are given along with **antihypertensives**.
15. **Potassium salts** are given with thiazide diuretics.
16. **Ammonium chloride** is given with organomercurials.
17. **Water** is called **physiological/natural diuretic.**
18. Spironolactone is an **aldosterone antagonist**.
19. Acetazolamide inhibits the enzyme **carbonic anhydrase**.
20. Spironolactone is contraindicated in **Addison's disease**.

Chapter 10

Hormone and Hormone Antagonists

- Thyroid hormones
- Parathormone
- Vitamin D
- Oral hypoglycemic agents/oral antidiabetic agents
- Progesterone
- Corticosteroids (adrenocortical hormones)
- Antithyroid drugs
- Calcitonin (thyrocalcitonin)
- Insulin
- Estrogens
- Oxytocin

A. THYROID HORMONES

Q 1. Define hormone and hormone antagonists.

Hormone

Hormones are chemical messengers that transport a signal from one cell to another.

Hormone Antagonists

Hormone antagonists are a specific type of receptor antagonists which act upon hormone and block its action.

Q 2. Describe in brief about "thyroid hormones".

Thyroid Hormones

- Thyroid hormones significantly affect the metabolic activities of the body.
- Thyroxine (T4), Tri-iodothyronine (T3) and calcitonin are secreted by parafollicular cells of thyroid gland are naturally secreted hormones of thyroid gland.
- Levothyroxine is known as L-thyroxine which is a synthetic form of tri-iodothyronine.

1. Levothyroxine Sodium

- It is a hormone of choice for thyroid hormone replacement therapy because of its consistent potency and prolonged duration of action.
- It is almost completely absorbed from GIT but it takes 1–3 weeks from beginning of therapy, to get full effect.

Therapeutic use/Indication

It is used in the treatment of hypothyroidism.

Adverse Effects

- Anginal pain
- Arrhythmia
- Muscle cramp
- Tremors
- Diarrhoea, vomiting
- Flushing
- Sweating

Contraindications

Thyrotoxicosis

Dosage

Levothyroxine sodium tablet : 50–100 μg daily.

2. Liothyronine Sodium

- It has a quick onset of action.
- After SC administration the response appears within 4–6 hours and maximum response is seen in 2 days.
- Its half life is about 8 days.

B. ANTITHYROID DRUGS

Q 1. Define and classify antithyroid drugs. Give an account of antithyroid agents.

Antithyroid Drugs

The drugs which prevent biosynthesis of thyroid hormones and are used in the treatment of thyrotoxicosis are called antithyroid drugs.

Classification

1. Iodine and iodides, e.g. radioiodine, iodine.
2. Thiouracil compounds, e.g. propylthiouracil, methylthiouracil, carbimazole, methimazole.
3. Aromatic amines and phenols, e.g. sulphaguanidine, PAS.
4. Lithium salts, e.g. lithium carbonate.
5. Miscellaneous, e.g. potassium perchlorate, potassium thiocyanate.

1. Thiouracil Compounds

- Thiourea and the related thiouracil compounds considerably decrease the thyroid hormones.
- These drugs are rapidly absorbed from the gut and widely circulated in the body and excreted via the urine.
- *Examples:* Propylthiouracil, methylthiouracil, carbimazole, methimazole.
- Thiouracil compounds inhibit the formation of thyroid hormone through inhibiting the oxidation of iodine to iodine by peroxide enzyme and blocking the coupling of iodothyrosines to form iodothyronines.
- **Propylthiouracil:** It is a thiouracil compound.

Therapeutic uses/Indications

i. It is used in the treatment of thyrotoxicosis ii. In hyperthyroidism

Adverse Effects

- Drug fever
- Skin rash
- Agranulocytosis

Contraindications

- Pregnant and lactating women
- Hepatic and renal impairment

Dosage

Propylthiouracil tablet : 300–600 mg daily orally.

Brand Name: Propacil.

2. Iodine

- Iodides act through inhibition of the protease enzyme which release T_3 and T_4 from thyroglobulin.
- Iodine is usually given as tablets of potassium iodide.

Use: In the treatment of thyrotoxicosis (preoperative treatment).

Contraindication: Breastfeeding.

Adverse effects: Headache, bronchitis, insomnia.

Dosage: Potassium iodide tab 60–80 mg daily.

3. Radioactive Iodine (I^{131}, I^{132})

Radioactive iodine emits mainly β-rays with a small γ-component and destroy thyroid tissue.

Use: It is mainly used to treat hyperthyroidism and thyroid carcinoma.

Adverse effects: Hypothyroidism.

Contraindications: Pregnancy and lactation.

4. Potassium Perchlorate

- Perchlorates act by blocking the uptake of iodide by the thyroid. It has the risk of aplastic anemia, therefore no longer used in the treatment or hyperthyrodism.

C. PARATHORMONE

Q 1. What is parathormone? Describe in brief parathormone.

Parathormone (Parathyroid Hormone) (PTH)

- Parathormone is a hormone secreted by the chief cells of parathyroid glands.
- Parathormone controls serum calcium level through its effect on bone, kidney and intestine.
- It helps the body to store and use calcium by increasing its absorption from intestine, release of calcium from bones into blood and conservation of calcium by the kidneys.

Mechanism of Action

Parathormone increases the ionic calcium of plasma and extracellular fluid. This effect is produced by following mechanisms:

1. Mobilization of calcium present in the bone. There is reabsorption of calcium and phosphorus from bone into the extracellular fluid.
2. Increased reabsorption of calcium by the renal tubules.
3. Increased absorption of calcium from the gut.
4. A fall in plasma calcium level stimulates the secretion of parathormone and a rise in plasma calcium level inhibits the secretion of parathormone.

Therapeutic uses/Indications

1. To control hypocalcemia and anaphylactic reaction.
2. In the diagnosis of pseudohypoparathyroidism.

Adverse Reactions

Hypercalcemia, kidney stones, tiredness, muscle fatigue, abdominal pains, constipation.

Contraindication

Hypercalcemia

Q 2. What do you mean by hypoparathyroidism? Explain calcitriol.

Hypoparathyroidism

It is the condition in which their is a low secretion of parathyroid hormone (PTH) from parathyroid gland.

Signs and Symptoms

- Hypocalcemia
- Tingling or burning in fingertips, toes and lips
- Muscle aches
- Muscle cramps
- Weakness
- Fatigue
- Painful menstrual periods

Treatment

Treatment of hypoparathyroidism includes administration of activated vitamin D (calcitriol) and calcium supplements.

Calcitriol

- It is active form of vitamin D, chemically it is 1, 25-dihydroxycholecalciferol.
- It is used to treat and prevent low level of calcium and bone disease in patients whose kidneys and parathyroid glands are not working normally.

Uses/Indications

1. Used in patient with kidney disease shows vitamin D deficiency.
2. It is used to treat calcium/phosphorus imbalance especially associated with hypoparathyroidism.

Dosage

Calcitriol capsule : 0.25 μg orally twice daily.

Brand Names

Rocaltrol, Calcijex.

D. CALCITONIN (THYROCALCITONIN)

Q 1. Describe in brief calcitonin/thyrocalcitonin).

Calcitonin/Thyrocalcitonin

- Calcitonin is a hormone produced and released by the C cells of thyroid glands.
- Calcitonin is a polypeptide containing 32 amino acids.
- Calcitonin decreases the plasma calcium concentration.

Mechanism of Action

Calcitonin lowers the plasma calcium level. This effect is produced by blocking parathyroid hormone induced bone reabsorption. It also increases the excretion of calcium in the urine. Calcitonin is secreted in response to increase in the calcium level of plasma.

Therapeutic uses

1. Used to treat hypercalcemia caused by hyperparathyroidism.
2. To relieve bone pain.

Dosage

Calcitonin injection 100 IU/day by SC or IM

Brand Names

Miacalcin, Zycalcit.

Adverse Effects

- Blurred vision
- Chills or fever
- Difficulty in breathing and swallowing
- Frequent urination
- Muscle aches and pains
- Muscle cramps in hand, arms, feet, legs.

Contraindications

- Cancer
- Low vitamin D levels
- Low amount of calcium in the blood.

E. VITAMIN D

Q 1. Write a note on vitamin D/calciferol.

Vitamin D

- Vitamin D is also called calciferol or cholecalciferol.
- Vitamin D is actually a hormone rather than vitamin.
- Vitamin D is the name applied to two related fat-soluble substances:
  1. Cholecalciferol (vitamin D_3)
  2. Ergocalciferol (vitamin D_2)
- Vitamin D_3 is obtained from ergosterol.
- Vitamin D_2 is obtained from 7-dehydrocholesterol.
- Vitamin D_3 is also called sunshine as it is obtained by the action of sun's UV rays on the sterols present in the skin.
- Sources of vitamin D are cod liver oil, butter, milk, yeast, ghee, halinut liver oil.
- Vitamin D is an essential nutrient for the body and is useful to absorb calcium.
- Ergocalciferol (vitamin D_2) is a representative vitamin D compound.

Ergocalciferol (Vitamin D_2)

Ergocalciferol is obtained by exposing ergosterol to ultraviolet light for the proper length of time.

Therapeutic uses/Indications

1. To prevent vitamin D deficiency caused by malabsorption or chronic liver disease.
2. In the treatment of rickets.
3. In the management of hypocalcemia and hypoparathyroidism.

Adverse Effects

- Anorexia
- Lassitude
- Nausea, vomiting, diarrhoea
- Weight loss
- Polyuria
- Headache, vertigo

Contraindications

- Renal insufficiency
- Hyperphosphatemia
- Hypercalcemia
- Metastatic calcification

Dosage

Ergocalciferol tablet : 1.25 mg (50000 units), daily for limited period.

F. INSULIN

Q 1. Describe "insulin" as an antidiabetic agent/hypoglycemic agent/ parenteral hypoglycemic agent.

Insulin

- Insulin is a polypeptide hormone secreted by β cells of the islets of Langerhans of pancreas.
- The commercial sourced insulin is the pancreas of ox and pig.
- Deficiency of insulin synthesis and secretion lead to diabetes mellitus.

Mechanism of Action

1. Insulin enhances the conversion of glucose to glycogen in skeletal muscle.
2. Insulin inhibits the conversion of glucose from fats, proteins and amino acids.

Role of Insulin in Diabetes Mellitus

The diabetic syndrome is due to a relative or absolute deficiency of insulin and is characterized by a rise in blood glucose. Hyperglycemia causes glycosuria with consequent osmotic diuresis and electrolyte and water depletion.

The symptoms of diabetes mellitus are polyuria, glycosuria, loss of weight and ketosis.

Insulin is used mainly to treat diabetes mellitus but may also stimulate appetite.

Adverse Effects

- Hypoglycemia
- Hypersensitivity
- Lipomata and fat atrophy at the site of repeated injection

Contraindications

- Hypoglycemia
- Hypokalemia
- Hepatic disease
- Renal failure

Therapeutic uses

1. To control diabetes mellitus.
2. To treat hyperkalemia.
3. To treat severe ketosis or diabetic coma.
4. To control diabetes in pregnancy, during surgery and infection.
5. Used to control IDDM, NIDDM, diabetes.

Classification

a. Short-acting insulins, e.g. plain insulin, insulin zinc suspension.

b. Intermediate-acting insulins, e.g. globulin zinc insulins, insulin zinc suspension (lente).

c. Long-acting insulins, e.g. protamine zinc insulins, insulin zinc suspension (ultra lente).

Preparations

i. ***Insulin IP (soluble insulin):*** It is an aqueous solution of crystalline insulin. It may be administered subcutaneously, intramuscularly or intravenously. It has onset action about 30 minutes, duration of action 6–8 hours.

ii. ***Zinc insulin suspensions:*** Insulin zinc preparations are suspensions of insulin with zinc chloride. These insulin zinc suspensions are also known as lente insulins. They are available as containing 40 units, 80 units per ml.

   a. *Insulin zinc suspension (amorphous) insulin semilente:* This insulin has onset action 1 hour, duration of action 12–16 hours.

   b. *Insulin zinc suspension (insulin lente):* It is a mixture of amorphous and crystalline forms. Insulin lente has onset action 2–4 hours, duration of action 18–32 hours.

   c. *Insulin zinc supension (crystalline) IP (insulin ultralente):* It has an onset of action 6–8 hours and duration of action 36 hours.

iii. ***Protamine zinc insulin:*** This is a suspension of insulin zinc chloride and protamine. It has onset action 3–6 hours and duration of action 24–48 hours. Hypersensitivity reaction may occur.

iv. ***Globulin zinc insulin:*** The globulin zinc insulin has intermediate duration of action 12–16 hours. These preparations are little used.

Q 2. Why insulin is not given/administered orally?

i. Insulin is a polypeptide hormone secreted by β cells of the islets of Langerhans.

ii. Commercially it is available as a mixture of hormone extracted from pancreas of cattle (bovine) or pigs.

iii. When insulin is administered orally, proteolytic enzymes and gastric juice cause its degradation.

iv. So, no therapeutic response is obtained in diabetes mellitus. Therefore, insulin is not given orally.

Q 3. Give the differences between:
a. IDDM (Type I) and NIDDM (Type II)
b. Diabetes mellitus and diabetes insipidus
c. Hyperglycemia and hypoglycemia.

a. *IDDM (Type I diabetes)*	*NIDDM (Type II diabetes)*
1. Onset is less than 20 years	1. Onset is more than 30 years
2. Normal weight individual	2. Obese individual
3. Severe insulin deficiency	3. Moderate insulin deficiency
4. Ketoacidosis is common	4. Ketoacidosis is rare
5. β cell depletion	5. Mild β cell depletion
6. Hyperglycemia controls with insulin	6. Hyperglycemia controls with oral hypoglycaemic drugs

b. *Diabetes mellitus*	*Diabetes insipidus*
1. It is due to deficiency of insulin	1. It is due to deficiency of ADH (anti-diuretic hormone)
2. It is disorder of pancreas	2. It is disorder of posterior pituitary gland
3. Blood sugar level becomes high and glucose appears in urine	3. Blood sugar level is normal and glucose does not appear in urine
4. There is high level of blood cholesterol and ketone bodies formation	4. No formation of ketone bodies
5. Symptoms are excessive thirst, excessive urine production, excessive eating (excess appetite)	5. Symptoms are excretion of large quantity of urine, thirst and dehydration

c. *Hyperglycemia*	*Hypoglycemia*
1. It is due to deficiency of insulin	1. It is due to excess of insulin
2. Blood sugar level is raised	2. Blood sugar level is low
3. Symptoms are loss of weight, tiredness, sweating, irritability and double vision, weak eyesight	3. Symptoms are excessive hunger due to break down of muscle tissues

Q 4. Write a note on "diabetes mellitus". Mention the drugs used in diabetes mellitus.

Diabetes Mellitus

- Diabetes mellitus is a condition caused due to raised glucose concentration in the blood due to deficiency of insulin.
- Diabetes is a group of diseases characterized by a state of chronic hyperglycemia.
- The hyposecretion of insulin from the β cells of islets of Langerhans leads to increased blood sugar level. The sugar passes through urine, the condition is called diabetes mellitus.

- The "diabetes" means large volume of urine is passed. The term "mellitus" means sweet.
- In diabetes mellitus the blood glucose level exceeds normal renal threshold level (180/100 ml) hence glucose is found in the urine.

Types

- ***Type 1. Insulin dependent diabetes mellitus (IDDM):***
  - It is also called Juvenile-onset diabetes mellitus.
  - It occurs in children and adolescents.
- ***Type 2. Non-insulin dependent diabetes mellitus (NIDDM):***
  - It is also called maturity onset diabetes mellitus.
  - It develops in middle ages or in elderly patients who are often obese.
- ***Type 3. Malnutrition-related diabetes mellitus (MRDM):***
- ***Type 4. Secondary diabetes:*** It may be due to certain pancreatic disorders or genetic syndrome or may be drug-induced.

Signs and Symptoms of Diabetes Mellitus

Excessive thirst, excessive urination, fatigue, dryness of mouth, weight loss.

Drugs used in Diabetes Mellitus

Insulin, glibenclamide, tolbutamide, phenformin, metformin, chlorpropamide.

Q 5. What are hypoglycemic agents? Classify hypoglycemic agents with suitable examples.

Hypoglycemic Agents/Antidiabetic Agents

The drugs which lower the blood sugar level and are used in the treatment of diabetes mellitus are known as hypoglycemic agents.

Classification

- Hormones (parenteral): Insulin and its derivatives.
- Oral hypoglycemic agents.
  i. Sulphonyl urea derivatives, e.g. chlorpropamide, tolbutamide, glibenclamide.
  ii. Biguanide derivatives, e.g. phenformin, metformin.
- Plant source, e.g. guar gum.

G. ORAL HYPOGLYCEMIC AGENTS/ORAL ANTIDIABETIC AGENTS

Q 1. Define and classify oral hypoglycemic agents.

Oral Hypoglycemic Agents

Oral hypoglycemic drugs lower blood glucose levels. These drugs are effective orally. To control diabetes, the main drawback of insulin is that it is not effective orally and must be administered by injection.

Classification

i. ***Sulfonylureas:***

First generation drugs: (i) Tolbutamide, (ii) chlorpropamide.

Second generation drugs: Glibenclamide, glipizide, gliclazide, glimepride.

ii. ***Biguanides:*** Metformin, phenformin.

iii. ***Meglitinide:*** Repaglinide, nepaglinide.

iv. ***Thiazolidinediones:*** Rosiglitazone, pioglitazone.

v. ***α-Glucosidase inhibitors:*** Acarbose, miglitol.

v. ***Plant source:*** Agar-agar.

Q 2. Explain sulphonylurea derivatives as a hypoglycemic agents?

Sulphonylurea Derivatives

Sulphonylureas are used therapeutically to cause hypoglycemia.

Mechanism of Action

The sulphonylureas stimulate pancreatic β cells to produce greater amount of insulin and inhibit the output of glucose from the liver.

Examples: Glibenclamide, tolbutamide, chlorpropamide.

1. Glibenclamide

- It is a long-acting sulphonylurea.
- It may occasionally show hypoglycemia 4 hours or more after food and may be dose related.
- As it stimulates appetite, it increases body weight which is main disadvantage.

Uses

1. In the treatment of diabetes mellitus. 2. As a hypoglycemic agent.

Adverse Effects

- GI disturbances
- Headache
- Liver disorders
- Exfoliative dermatitis
- Hypoglycemia

Contraindications

- Ketoacidosis
- Porphyria
- Pregnancy and breastfeeding

Dosage

Glibenclamide tablet : 2.5–15 mg daily orally in divided doses.

Brand Names

Daonil, Euglucon.

2. Tolbutamide

It is a sulfonylurea derivative.

Mechanism of Action

Tolbutamide activates functioning of β cells in pancreas to release insulin, decrease blood sugar level.

Therapeutic use

In diabetes mellitus.

Adverse Effects

- Joint pains
- Hypoglycemia
- Skin rash, urticaria, nausea, heartburn
- Eczema, dizziness, vertigo
- Headache, weakness
- Leukopenia, aplastic anemia

Contraindications

- Hypersensitivity
- Diabetic coma
- Ketoacidosis
- Pregnancy and lactation

Dosage

Tolbutamide tablet : 1 gm daily after meal up to 3 gm daily.

Brand Name

Rastinon.

3. Chlorpropamide

- It is a sulphonylurea derivative.
- It acts by stimulating β cells of the pancreas to release insulin.

Uses

1. As a oral hypoglycemic agent
2. For the treatment of NIDDM

Adverse Effects

- Nausea, vomiting
- Loss of appetite, hunger
- Dizziness
- Itching

Contraindications

- Hypoglycemia
- Pituitary hormone deficiency
- Hepatic porphyria

Dosage

Chlorpropamide tablet : 100–500 mg once daily.

Brand Names

Diabenese, Diabetol, Diabetin.

Q 3. Write a note on "biguanides" as hypoglycemic agents.

Biguanides

These drugs stimulate the peripheral utilization of glucose.

1. Phenformin

It is an oral biguanide antidiabetic agent.

Adverse Effects

- Anorexia, nausea, vomiting, diarrhoea
- Metallic taste in mouth
- Weight loss
- Acute pancreatitis

Contraindications

- Hypersensitivity
- Alcoholism
- Hepatic and renal damage
- Pregnancy

Dosage

- Phenformin tablet : 25 mg, 1–4 times daily orally.

Brand Names

DBI, Asoformin.

2. Metformin

It is an oral biguanide derivative used as hypoglycemic agent.

Mechanism of Action

It inhibits hepatic glucose production, increases senstivity of peripheral tissue to insulin.

Therapeutic uses

1. As hypoglycemic agent.
2. Used as first-line medication for the treatment of type 2 diabetes.
3. To treat non-insulin dependent diabetes mellitus.
4. To treat insulin dependent diabetes mellitus in combination with insulin.
5. To treat diabetes associated with hyperlipoproteinaemia.

Adverse Effects

- Skin rash, vomiting, diarrhoea, nausea
- Drowsiness, tinnitus, vertigo
- Lactic acidosis
- Metallic taste in mouth
- Anorexia
- Thrombocytopenia

Contraindications

- Hypersensitivity
- Alcoholism
- Hepatic renal damage
- Pregnancy

H. OESTROGENS

Q 1. Write in brief about "oestrogens".

Estrogens

- Oestradiol, oestrone and oestriol are naturally occurring oestrogens.
- They secreted by the ovary, placenta, adrenal cortex and testes.
- They are metabolised particularly in the liver and excreted in the urine as glucuronides and sulphates.
- The oestrogens are feminising and are responsible for the normal development and maintenance of female genital tract and secondary sex characteristics.
- The oestrogens are mainly responsible for the maintenanace of the proliferative phase of the endometrium during the menstrual cycle and together with progesterone, the secretory phase.
- Examples of synthetic oestrogens: Dienestrol, hexoestrol, methallenestril, chlorotrianisene.

Therapeutic uses

1. In correction of menopausal syndrome
2. To treat amenorrhoea
3. To inhibit lactation
4. To treat breast cancer
5. To treat genital problems

1. Ethinylestradiol

- It is a representative estrogen.
- Ethinylestradiol is an estrogen medication which is used in birth control pills in combination with progestins.
- It works by stopping a woman's egg from fully developing each month.

Therapeutics uses

1. To treat menopausal symptoms.
2. Used to prevent pregnancy in combination with drospirenone.
3. To treat menstrual syndromes.
4. To treat gynaecological disorders.
5. In prophylaxis of osteoporosis.
6. Palliation in breast cancer in men and post-menopausal women.
7. Contraception in combination with progestogen.

Adverse Effects

- Nausea, vomiting, headache
- Abdominal cramps/bloating
- Breast tenderness
- Swelling of the ankles/feet

Contraindications

- Pregnancy
- Estrogen dependent cancer
- Thrombophlebitis
- Thromboembolic disorders

Dosage

Ethinylestradiol tablet : 10–20 μg daily orally.

Brand Names

Ovral, Ogestrel, Bandhan.

2. Cloniphene Citrate

- It is a synthetic nonsteroidal drug.
- It is readily absorbed orally and largely metabolised in the liver and excreted via the bile into gut.
- It has a weak oestrogenic action but also has some powerful antioestrogenic properties.
- It induces ovulation in an ovulatory women and regulates irregular ovulation.

I. PROGESTERONE

Q 1. Write in brief about progesterone (progestogens).

Progesterone

- Progesterone is a natural occurring progestogen hormone, synthesized by placenta, adrenal cortex, testis.
- It is less effective orally due to complete metabolism by liver, so it is given by intramuscular route.
- It is also given in the form of implant.

Mechanism of Action

a. ***On ovary:*** Inhibition of ovulation.

b. ***On uterus:*** Converts endometrium for secretory phase and makes the myometrium less sensitive to oxytocin. It also causes relaxation of the uterus in late pregnancy.

Synthetic/Semi-synthetic Substitutes

1. Medroxyprogesterone acetate
2. Ethisterone
3. Norethisterone
4. Levonorgestrel

Therapeutic uses

1. Hormonal contraception
2. In functional uterine bleeding
3. In dysmennorrhoea
4. In ammenorrhoea
5. In endometrial carcinoma
6. In premenstrual tension

1. Medroxyprogesterone Acetate

It is a complementary progestogenic drug.

Uses/Indications

1. In endometriosis dysfunctional uterine bleeding.
2. To treat secondary ammenorrhoea.
3. An adjunct in hormone replacement therapy.

Contraindications

1. Pregnancy
2. Genital neoplasm
3. Hepatic impairment
4. Porphyria

Use

It is used in the treatment on infertility in women caused by disorder of ovulation.

Adverse Effects

- Flushing (feeling of warmth)
- Stomach upsets
- Headache, vomiting
- Breast discomfort

Contraindications

- Hypersensitivity
- Breastfeeding
- Abnormal uterine bleeding

Dosage

Clomiphene tablets : 50 mg orally for 5 days from cycle day 3 to cycle day 7.

Brand Names

Clomid, Serophene.

Dosage

Medroxyprogesterone acetate tablet : 5 mg.

Dose

For mild to moderate endometriosis: 10 mg 3 times daily for 90 days, beginning on first day of cycle.

For dysfunctional uterine bleeding: 2.5–10 mg daily for 5–10 days; beginning on day 16–21 of cycle for 2 cycles.

For secondary amenorrhoea: 2.5–10 mg daily for 5–10 days, beginning on day 16–21 of cycle for 3 cycles.

Brand Names

Provera 104, Depo-Provera.

2. Norethisterone

Norethisterone is also known as norethidrone and is used as birth control pills. Menopausal hormone therapy and for the treatment of gynaecological disorders.

Uses/Indications

1. In endometriosis
2. In menorrhagia
3. In severe dysmenorrhoea
4. In contraception

Adverse Effects

- Irregular vaginal bleeding
- Changes in menstrual flow
- Breast tenderness
- Nausea, vomiting
- Bloating
- Weight changes

Contraindications

- Pregnancy
- Undiagnosed vaginal bleeding
- Hepatic impairment

Dosage

Norethisterone tablet : 5 mg.

Dose

For endometriosis: 10 mg daily starting on fifth day of cycle.
For menorrhagia: 5 mg, three times daily for 10 days to stop bleeding to prevent bleeding 5 mg, twice daily from day 19–26 of cycle.
For dysmenorrhoea: 5 mg, 2–3 times daily from day 5–24 for 3–4 cycles.

Brand Name

Progestin.

Q 2. Write a note on "oral contraceptives/oral pills".

Oral Contraceptives

Contraceptives: *Contraceptives are drugs which prevent conception.* These drugs control fertility so are also called antifertility drugs.

These contraceptive drugs suppress fertility at will for a desired period with complete return of fertility on discontinuation of oral contraceptive drugs.

Fertility control by drug: The drugs control fertility by following mechanism:

a. By inhibiting ovulation in females.
b. By inhibiting spermatogenesis in males.
c. By decreasing rate of egg transport.
d. By preventing maturation of ovum.
e. The drugs change the cervical mucus which inhibits sperms penetration in the ovum.
f. The drugs interfere with the implantation of fertilized ovum.

Types

The oral contraceptive preparations are:

i. Progestins alone
ii. Combination of oestrogen and progestins.
iii. Oestrogen alone followed by oestrogen + progestin combination.

Method of Administration

1. ***Combination method:*** The oestrogen and progestin is administered from 5th day to 25th day of menstrual cycle.
2. ***Sequential method:*** Oestrogen alone is administered alone and is given from 5th day to 20th day, from 21st day to 25th day oestrogen + progestin combination is administered.

Mechanism of Action

In the combination method FSH rises and LH peak concentration is suppressed due to which follicular growth is decreased. This prevents ovulation.

In sequential method, the oestrogen given suppresses FSH secretions on the contrary stimulates LH secretion. This unusual rise of LH suppresses early follicle stimulating hormones rise due to which growth of follicle is reduced and ovulation formation is prevented.

Pharmacological Actions

Action on ovaries: The combined drugs and sequential drugs depress function of ovaries. The follicular development is decreased. In ovulating women morphological changes are not observed.

Endometrial change: The endometrial change varies with the preparation used as contraceptive.

1. With combination of drugs estrogens and progestins, there is stromal deciduation towards end of the menstrual cycle.
2. There is no change with sequential drugs. Progestational effect on glandular tissue is seen during the last 5 days of cycle.
3. There may be increase in transcortin (cortisol binding protein).
4. These contraceptive drugs may cause hyperglycemia, glycosuria, hypertension.
5. There may be increased in thyroxine binding globulin.

Side Effects/Adverse Effects

- Nausea, vomiting, anorexia
- Weight gain
- Fluid retention
- Breast enlargement
- Hypertension
- Carcinogenicity

Preparations

Brand name	Drug combination
1. Anovlar 21	Ethinyl estradiol (0.05 mg) and norethisterone acetate (4 mg)
2. Primovlar 30	Ethinyl estradiol (0.03 mg) and norgestrel (0.15 mg)
3. Ovral	Ethinyl estradiol (0.05 mg) and norgestrel (0.5 mg)
4. Lyndiol 1	Ethinyl estradiol (0.05 mg) and lynestrenol (1 mg)

J. OXYTOCIN

Q 1. Give the short account of "oxytocin".

Oxytocin

- Oxytocin is a hormone secreted by posterior lobe of pituitary gland.
- Oxytocin is a polypeptide which contains 9 amino acids.
- Oxytocin is used to control postpartum haemorrhage.

Mechanism of Action

1. Oxytocin stimulates the uterus and produces contraction of uterus which helps in the easy expulsion of the foetus.
2. It also causes ejection of milk through contraction of the myoepithelial cells around the alveoli of the mammary glands.

Pharmacokinetics

Oxytocin is inactivated orally and absorbed rapidly after intramuscular administration. It can also be absorbed from nasal and buccal/membrane.

By IV route onset of action is 1 minute, duration of action is 30 minutes, plasma half life is 12–17 minutes.

Pharmacological Actions

1. ***On uterus:*** In humans, a small dose of oxytocin gives increase the tone and amplitude of contraction. Large doses produce tonic contractions, there may be uterine rupture, water retention and foetal asphyxiation. Oxytocin causes fundus to contract while to cervix dilates, this helps in easy expulsion of the foetus. Oxytocin is used for induction of labour.
2. ***On mammary gland:*** Oxytocin stimulates the myoepithelium and helps in increasing expulsion of milk from mammary gland.
   Oxytocin is ineffective when given orally. The absorption is rapid on intramuscular injection. The oxytocinase present in blood plasma, placenta of pregnant women and uterine tissue inactivates oxytocin.
3. ***Action on kidneys:*** Oxytocin in large dose causes decrease in urine output. Pulmonary oedema occurs if large quantity of intravenous fluids and oxytocin are administered together. The conventional doses of oxytocin do not cause any adverse effect.

4. ***Action on heart (CVS):*** The normal doses (conventional doses) used in induction of labour cause no effect on blood pressure. Large doses cause vasodilatation causing fall in blood pressure, flushing and reflex tachycardia.

Therapeutic uses

i. Oxytocin is used in the induction of labour.
ii. Used to control postpartum haemorrhage.
iii. To promote milk ejection it is given as intranasal spray few minutes before suckling. Oxytocin does not increase milk production. It is used to stimulate milk release.
iv. It is used to induce abortion during 2nd to 3rd trimesters.

Adverse Effects

- Hypotension
- Increased pulse rate
- Jaundice
- Anorexia, vomiting, nausea
- Constipation
- Skin rash
- Asphyxia, hypoxia

Contraindications

- Hypersensitivity
- Foetal distress
- Serum toxemia
- Hypertonic uterine contractions

Dosage

Oxytocin injection 10 units/ml.

Dose

For induction of labour: By IV infusion initially 0.001–0.002 units/minute, increased in 0.001–0.002 units/minute, increments at intervals of 30 minutes. Until maximum of 3–4 contractions occur every 10 minutes.

For prevention of postpartum haemorrhage: By slow IV injection 5 units immediately after birth or 10 units by IM injection immediate after birth.

For treatment of postpartum haemorrhage: By slow IV injection 10 units immediately after birth.

Brand Name

Pitocin.

K. CORTICOSTEROIDS (ADRENOCORTICAL HORMONES)

Q 1. Write a note on "corticosteroids"/"adrenocortical hormones".

Corticosteroids/Adrenocortical Hormones

- Corticosteroids are the hormones secreted by adrenal cortex.
- Corticosteroids control the metabolism of carbohydrates, proteins, fats and water/electrolytes.

Adenocortical hormones are classified into:

a. Glucocorticoid	: Cortisone
	: Hydrocortisone (cortisol)
b. Mineralocorticoid	: Aldosterone
	: Desoxycorticosterone
c. Sex hormone	: Estrogen
	: Androgen

Glucocorticoids

The important glucorticoid secreted in man is hydrocortisone. It possesses some mineralocorticoid activity as well. Cortisone is less potent and is converted to hydrocortisone by liver.

They are classified as:

1. Short acting, e.g. cortisone, hydrocortisone
2. Intermediate acting, e.g. prednisolone, triamcinolone
3. Long acting, e.g. dexamethasone, betamethasone.

Side Effects

- Weight gain
- Edema and hypokalemia
- Hyperglycemia
- Osteoporosis
- Psychiatric disturbance
- Peptic ulceration
- Cushing syndrome
- Retarded growth

Contraindications

- In peptic ulcer
- Active tuberculosis
- Diabetes mellitus
- Psychosis
- Pregnancy

Therapeutic uses

1. ***Replacement therapy:*** Adrenal insufficiency can result from structural or functional lesions of adrenal cortex. In all such insufficiencies corticosteroids are indicated.
2. ***Rheumatic disorders:*** Corticosteroids are widely used in the treatment of rheumatic disorders.

3. ***Renal diseases:*** In nephrotic syndromes glucocorticoids are the first line treatment.
4. ***Allergic diseases:*** Allergic manifestations of limited duration can be treated well using glucocorticoids.
5. ***Bronchial asthma and other pulmonary disorders:*** Corticosteroids are frequently used in conditions such as asthma and COPD.
6. ***Infectious diseases:*** Use of corticosteroids in AIDS patients with *Pneumocystis carinii* pneumonia is beneficial.
7. ***Ocular diseases:*** Glucocorticoids suppress inflammation in the eye and can preserve sight when used properly.
8. ***Skin diseases:*** Glucocorticoids are quite useful in variety of inflammatory dermatoses.
9. ***Gastrointestinal diseases:*** In certain diseases like inflammatory bowel disease (chronic ulcerative colitis, Crohn's disease), glucocorticoids are beneficial.
10. ***Hepatic diseases:*** In autoimmune hepatitis prednisone plays beneficial role.
11. ***Malignancies:*** Glucocorticoids are one component of combination chemotherapy for malignancies.
12. ***Miscellaneous uses:*** In the treatment of conditions such as thrombocytopenia, autoimmune destruction of erythrocytes, organ transplantation and spinal cord injury.

Q 2. Write in brief about "hydrocortisone".

Hydrocortisone

- Hydrocortisone is a glucocorticoid.
- It is also known as cortisol.
- It is the treatment of choice for adrenocortical insufficiency.

Therapeutic uses/Indications

1. Used in adrenocortical insufficiency.
2. Used in anaphylactic shock.
3. Used in inflammatory bowel disease.
4. Used in asthma.
5. Used in skin disorders (redness, swelling, itching).

Adverse Effects

- Dyspepsia, peptic ulceration
- Abdominal distension
- Osteoporosis, bone fracture
- Euphoria, depression, psychosis, insomnia
- Myocardial infarction, thromboembolism

Contraindications

Systemic infection.

Dosage

20–30 mg daily in divided doses orally.

Brand Names

Wycort, Sotra-cort.

Objective Questions with Answers in Bold Letters

1. The stimulation of **H_1 receptors** enhances secretion of hydrochloric acid in the stomach.
2. **Hormones** are the chemical messengers that convey information from one cell to the next.
3. Iodine acts through inhibition of **protease enzyme.**
4. Parathormone controls **serum calcium** level.
5. Calcitonin is a polypeptide containing **32** amino acids.
6. Calcitonin is a hormone produced and released by the **C cells** of thyroid gland.
7. **Vitamin D** is known as cholecalciferol.
8. **Vitamin D** is used in the treatment of **rickets.**
9. Deficiency of **insulin** leads to diabetes mellitus.
10. **Insulin** enhances the conversion of glucose to glycogen in skeletal muscle.
11. **Hypoglycemia** is adverse effect of insulin.
12. Protamine zinc insulin is a **long-acting insulin.**
13. **Insulin** is not administered orally.
14. IDDM means **insulin dependent diabetes mellitus.**
15. NIDDM means **non-insulin dependent diabetes mellitus.**
16. Diabetes insipidus is caused due to deficiency of **ADH.**
17. The drugs which lower excessive sugar level to normal level are called **hypoglycemic** agents.
18. Insulin is a **parenteral** hypoglycemic agent.
19. Phenformin and metformin are **biguanide** type of oral hypoglycemic agent.
20. Glibenclamide is **sulphonylurea** type of antidiabetic agent.
21. Biguanide drugs stimulate the peripheral **utilization of glucose**.
22. Oxytocin is used to **control postpartum haemorrhage**.
23. Oxytocin is a polypeptide which contains **9 amino acids**.
24. Oxytocin enhances process of **parturition**.
25. Pictocin is a popular brand name of **oxytocin.**
26. **Hydrocortisone** is a main glucocorticoid.
27. **Aldosterone** is a main mineralocorticoid.
28. **Calcitriol** is used in the treatment of hypothyroidism.
29. **Calcitonin** is used to treat hypercalcemia.
30. **Insulin** is a polypeptide hormone produced by β cells in the pancreatic islets of Langerhans.

Chapter 11

Autocoids

Q 1. Define autocoids. Give classification.

The substances which have self-regulating power in the body are called autocoids.

Classification

1. Endogenous amines, e.g. histamine, 5-hydroxytryptamine (serotonin) (5-HT).
2. Polypeptides, e.g. bradykinins, kinins, kallidin, angiotensin.
3. Lipids, e.g. prostaglandins, prostacyclins.

Q 2. Discuss physiological role of histamine and serotonin.

A. Role of Histamine in the Body

1. Histamine may play an important role in gastric secretion with hormone gastrin.
2. It also plays a part in tissue growth and repair.
3. It helps in antigen–antibody reaction.
4. It contracts all plain muscles including muscles of uterus, bronchi, intestine.
5. Intradermal injection of histamine produces "triple response".
6. Histamine dilates blood capillaries and thereby causing fall in BP.

B. Role of Serotonin (5-HT) in the Body

1. It gives constriction of peripheral blood vessels.
2. It has stimulant action on heart.
3. It stimulates smooth muscles.
4. It plays important role in neurohumoral transmission.

Q 3. Explain "triple response" produced by histamine.

Intradermal administration of 10–20 μg of histamine in man produces a characteristic effect described by Lewis as a "triple response".

The "triple response" consists of:

1. Reddening at the site of injection described as a 'flush'.
2. The flush is followed by development of bright 'flare', i.e. an irregular outline.
3. Development of localised edema ('wheal' which is due to escape of fluid from the capillary).

Q 4. Describe the functions, pharmacological actions, receptors of histamine.

Or

Write a note on histamine.

Histamine

- Histamine is a potent biogenic amine.
- Histamine is released in many allergic states due to antigen–antibody reactions.
- Injection of histamine produces many of the allergic or anaphylactic symptoms such as wheal, urticaria, hypotension, bronchoconstriction.
- Histamine is derived from the amino acid histidine by the decarboxylation.

Storage and release: Histamine is stored in the mast cell of numerous sites, nose, mouth, and internal body surface and around the blood vessels. Non-mast cell histamine is found in the brain. It is released from the mast cell by various pathophysiological mechanism like when IgE antibodies are attached to the surface of mast cell and degranulate the mast cell.

Functions

1. Allergic response
2. Immediate hypersensitivity reactions
3. Acts as a neurotransmitter in the brain

Stimuli that Mediate Release of Histamine

1. Direct immunological release or antigen-mediated release
2. Indirect immunological release
   - Venoms
   - Radiation
   - Activation of anaphylatoxin
3. Non-antigen mediated or non-immunological release

Histamine Receptors

H_1 receptor: It is present on smooth muscle (bronchial muscle, intestinal muscle, blood vessels, CNS and endothelium)

It is worked by IP_3-DAG pathway.

H_2 receptor: It is present on cardiac muscle, mast cell and gastric parietal cell. It is worked by increasing cyclic-AMP.

H_3 receptor: It is present on brain, myenteric plexus. It is G-protein coupled receptor.

Pharmacological Actions

1. ***On blood vessels:*** Histamine produces constriction of large blood vessels. Histamine-induced headache is because of stretching of sensory nerve endings around the cranial nerves. Administration of histamine produces marked flushing in face and neck.
2. ***On blood pressure:*** In large dose histamine may produce prolonged hypotension.
3. ***Triple response:*** Intradermal injection of histamine shows three responses: a. Flush, b. flare, c. wheal.
4. ***On heart:*** Histamine increases amplitude of ventricular contraction. In high doses it produces ventricular arrhythmia.
5. ***On smooth muscles:*** Histamine directly stimulates the smooth muscles of various tissues including the bronchi and uterus. It may produce bronchospasm.
6. **Exocrine glands:** Histamine induces increase in gastric HCl secretion even in smaller doses. Histamine induces gastric acid secretion by parietal cells and pepsin secretion by chief cell stimulation.

Adverse Effects

- Hypotension
- Flushing
- Headache, diarrhoea
- Dyspnoea

Therapeutic/Clinical uses

1. To study gastric secretions.
2. In the diagnosis of leprosy.

Q 5. Define and classify antihistaminics with suitable examples.

Antihistaminics

The drugs which block the actions produced by histamine are called antihistaminics.

Classification

A. *H_1-receptor antagonists*

1. Aminoalkyl ether types, e.g. diphenhydramine, dimenhydrinate.
2. Alkylamine derivatives, e.g. chlorpheniramine, pheniramine.
3. Ethylene diamine derivatives, e.g. mepyramine, antazoline.
4. Piperazines, e.g. meclizine, buclizine, chlorcyclizine.
5. Phenothiazines, e.g. promethazine.

B. ***H_2-receptor antagonists:*** Reduce gastric acid secretion and prevent ulcers, e.g. cimetidine, ranitidine, famotidine, metiamide, burimamide.

Q 6. What are antihistaminics? Give the pharmacological actions, adverse effects, therapeutic uses and preparations of antihistaminics.

Antihistaminics

The drugs which block the action of histamine are called antihistaminics.

Pharmacological Actions

1. Antihistaminic Actions

Antihistaminic effectively antagonise the actions of injected histamine on smooth muscles.

Antihistaminics diminish the effect of histamine on other exocrine glands such as salivary and nasolacrimal glands.

2. Other Actions

a. *On CNS:* Antihistamines are normally sedative but cause excitement especially in overdose. They are used in the relief of motion sickness, in vomiting of early pregnancy and to reduce the rigidity and tremor of parkinsonism.

b. *Local anaesthetic and cardiodepressant actions:* Many antihistaminics are quite potent local anaesthetic, and cardiodepressant hence used in arrhythmias.

c. *Autonomic effect:* In higher concentration antihistamines may antagonise the actions of acetylcholine.
The atropine-like action can cause dry mouth and suppress nasopharyngeal secretions.

Adverse Effects

- Dizziness
- Tinitus
- Tremor
- Diplopia
- Incoordination
- Insomnia
- Teratogenicity is always a possibility in early pregnancy

Dosage of H_1 Antihistaminics

Drug	*Brand name*	*Dose*	*Route*
1. Diphenhydramine	Benadryl	25–50 mg t.i.d.	Oral
2. Mepyramine	Athisan	50–100 mg t.i.d.	Oral
3. Chlorpheniramine	Piriton	2–4 mg daily	Oral
4. Promethazine	Aromine	10 mg daily	Oral
5. Cuproheptadine	Ciplactin	4 mg t.i.d.	Oral

Q 7. Write a note on H_2-receptor antagonists/H_2-antihistaminics.

H_2-Receptor Antagonists/H_2-Antihistaminics

The drugs which block the actions of histamine on H_2-receptors by competitive inhibition are called H_2-receptor antagonists or H_2-antihistaminics. H_2-receptor antagonists reduce gastric acid secretion and prevent ulcers. For example:

i. Cimetidine
ii. Ranitidine
iii. Famotidine
iv. Metiamide
v. Burimamide

Cimetidine

It is a H_2-receptor antagonist.

Pharmacological Actions

Cimetidine markedly inhibits the basal and meal-stimulated gastric secretion.

On oral administration, cimetidine reduces the gastric secretion of acid to about 20% within an hour.

Adverse Effects

i. Skin rash
ii. Diarrhoea
iii. Muscle pain
iv. Hepatotoxicity
v. Sexual disturbances

Preparation and Dose

Cimetidine tablet IP

Dose: 200 mg twice daily orally

Trade Names

Cimetigate, Lock-2.

Therapeutic uses

i. In treatment of peptic ulcer.
ii. In treatment of duodenal ulcers.

Q 8. Write in brief about "5-HT receptor antagonists".

5-HT Receptor Antagonists

- These are also called serotonin receptor antagonists or serotonin receptor blockers.
- This class of medicines is used for the prevention and treatment of nausea and vomiting, particularly caused by chemotherapy, radiation therapy, etc.
- A number of selective antagonists for $5\text{-}HT_{2A/2C}$ and $5\text{-}HT_3$ receptors are currently available.

- Ketanserin is the prototype 5-HT_{2A} receptor antagonist.
- Large number of 5-HT_3 antagonist including ondansetron, dolasetron and granisetron are effective in the treatment of chemotherapy induced nausea.
- Examples of 5-HT receptor antagonits:
  1. Clozapine 2. Methysergide 3. Cyproheptadine

1. Clozapine

- It is a 5-$HT_{2A/2C}$ receptor antagonist represents a class of atypical anti-psychotic drug.
- Clozapine exerts its effects by blocking of 5-HT_{2A}/5-HT_{2C} serotonin receptors and D1–D4 dopamine receptors.

Adverse Effects

- Dizziness
- Light headedness
- Fainting

Uses/Indications

1. As antipsychotic
2. In dementia

Dosage

Clozapine tablet : 25–50 mg/day orally.

Brand Names

Clozaril, Fazaclo.

2. Methysergide

- It is an ergot derivative.
- It blocks 5-$HT_{2A/2C}$ receptors.

Uses

1. In migraine
2. In vascular headaches

Adverse Effects

- Seizures
- Ataxia
- Insomnia
- Lightheadedness
- Drowsiness

Dosage

Methysergide tablet : 4–8 mg daily.

Brand Names

Deseril, Sansert.

3. Cyproheptadine

It shows promient 5-HT_{2A} receptor antagonist activity.

Uses

It is used to control:

i. Red, irritated, itchy, watery eyes ii. Sneezing iii. Runny nose

Adverse Effects

- Mental disorders
- Confusion
- Mood changes
- Hallucinations
- Restlessness

Dosage

Cyproheptadine tablet : 4 mg orally every 8 hours.

Brand Names

Periactin, Cypon.

Q 9. Write a note on "prostaglandins".

Prostaglandin

- The prostaglandins are a group of physiologically active lipid compounds called eicosanoids having diverse hormone-like effect in animals.
- Prostaglandins have been found in almost every tissue in humans and other animals.
- They are derived enzymatically from the fatty acid arachidonic acid.
- Prostaglandins are grouped in six categories, i.e. A, B, C, D, E and F. Out of these PGE_2 and $PGE_{2\alpha}$ are used clinically.
- Prostaglandins were first discovered and isolated from human semen in 1930 by a Swedish Scientist 'Ulfvon Euler'.

Biosynthesis of Prostaglandins

- Prostaglandins are synthesized by oxidation of essential fatty acids (EFAs).
- γ-Linolenic acid (GLA), arachidonic acid (AA) and eicosapentaenoic acid (EiA) are essential fatty acids involved in the biosynthesis of prostaglandins.
- The activation of phospholipase A_2 by proinflammatory cytokines leads to a production of arachidonic acid from membrane phospholipids.
- Arachidonic acid gives rise to physiologically and pharmacologically active compounds known as prostaglandins (iG), thromboxanes (TX), leukotrienes (LT) and lipoxin (LX).
- Cyclooxygenase (COX) is the key enzyme in the synthesis of prostaglandins, prostacyclins and thromboxanes.
- Two isoforms of the COX enzyme have been characterized by:
  - Cyclooxygenase 1 (COX-1)
  - Cyclooxygenase 2 (COX-2)

- These two isoforms of COX are almost identical in structure but have important differences in substrate and inhibitor selectively.
- COX-1 is constitutively present in almost all tissues and produces protective PGs maintaining homeostasis in many organs (e.g. stomach, kidney), while COX-2 is induced by inflammatory stimuli and cytokines.

Schematic Representation of Biosynthesis of Prostaglandins

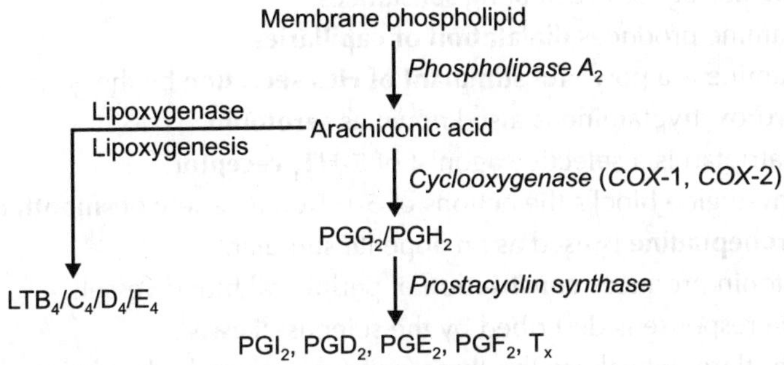

Mode of Action/Prostaglandin Receptor

Prostaglandins act or initiate pharmacological or physiological action by binding to specific receptors. There are currently ten known prostaglandin receptors on various cell types. All receptors are G-protein coupled receptors. **G-protein coupled receptors** are transmembrane receptors that sense molecules outside the cell and activate inside signal transduction pathways and ultimately cellular response. Below mentioned are all known receptors.

1. DP_{1-2} = DP_1, DP_2 receptor
2. EP_{1-4} = EP_1, EP_2, EP_3 and EP_4 receptors
3. FP = FP receptor
4. IP_{1-2} = IP_1 and IP_2 receptors
5. TP = TP receptor.

The names of the above receptors, corresponds to prostaglandins with which they bind, e.g. DP_{1-2} receptors bind to PGD_2.

Physiological Role/Pharmacological Functions of Prostaglandins

1. Prostaglandins activate inflammatory response, production of pain and fever.
2. Blood clots are formed when a blood vessel is damaged. A type of prostaglandin called thromboxane stimulates construction and clotting of platelets.

3. Some prostaglandins such as PGE_2 are involved in the induction of labour and other reproductive processes.
4. Prostaglandins are involved in several other organs such as gastrointestinal tract where they inhibit synthesis of acids and increases secretion of protective mucus also increases blood flow in kidney.

Objective Questions with Answers in Bold Letters

1. **Autocoids** are self-regulating substances.
2. Histamine produces **dialatation of capillaries.**
3. Histamine is a powerful **stimulant of HCl secretion** by the gastric mucosa.
4. 5-Hydroxytryptamine is also known as **serotonin.**
5. Sumatriptan is a selective agonist of **5-HT$_1$ receptor.**
6. Methysergide blocks the actions of 5-HT on a variety of **smooth muscles.**
7. **Cyproheptadine** is used as an appetite stimulant.
8. Serotonin produces **constriction** of peripheral blood vessels.
9. Triple response is described by the scientist **'Lewis'.**
10. Flush, flare, wheal are the three responses given by histamine are called **'triple response'.**
11. Histamine is a potent **biogenic amine.**
12. Histamine is released in many allergic states due to **antigen–antibody reactions.**
13. **H$_2$ receptors** are present in cardiac muscle, mast cells and gastric parietal cells.
14. Histamine induces gastric acid secretion may produce **peptic ulceration.**
15. Promethazine is a **H$_1$ receptor antagonist.**
16. **Benadryl** is a popular brand name of diphenhydramine.
17. Cimetidine, ranitidine and famotidine are **H$_2$ receptor antagonist.**
18. **Avomine** is a brand name of promethazine which is an antiemetic used in motion sickness.
19. Ondansetron is **5-HT$_3$ antagonist.**
20. Methysergide is used in the treatment of **migraine.**

Chapter 12

Chemotherapeutic Agents

- Penicillins
- Fluoroquinolones
- Sulphonamides
- Antiviral drugs
- Antimalarial drugs
- Cephalosporins
- Macrolides
- Antitubercular agents
- Antiamoebic drugs
- Antineoplastic agents
- Aminoglycosides
- Tetracyclines
- Antifungal drugs
- Anthelmintics (antiworms)

Introduction

1. ***Chemotherapy:*** Chemotherapy is defined as use of chemical compounds in the treatment of infectious disease so as to destroy microorganisms without damaging host tissue.
2. ***Chemotherapeutic agents:*** The agents which destroy or inhibit the growth of microorganisms without damaging host tissue, are known as chemotherapeutic agents.
3. ***Chemotherapeutic index:*** It is the ratio of maximum tolerated dose of a drug to its minimum curative dose.

$$\text{Chemotherapeutic index} = \frac{\text{maximum tolerated dose}}{\text{minimum curative dose}}$$

4. ***Bactericidals:*** The agents which kill or destroy the microorganisms are called bactericidal agents.
5. ***Bacteriostatics:*** The agents which stop or prevent growth of microorganisms are called bacteriostatics.
6. ***Antibiotics:*** Antibiotics are the chemical substances produced by microorganisms having the property of inhibiting the growth or destroying the microorganisms in high concentrations.

Q 1. Define and classify antibiotics giving suitable examples.

Antibiotics

Antibiotics are the chemical substances produced by microorganisms having the property of inhibiting the growth or destroying the microorganisms in high dilution.

Classification

1. Antibiotics mainly effective against gram +ve bacteria, e.g. penicillins, ampicillin, bacitracin, erythromycin.
2. Antibiotics mainly effective against gram –ve bacteria, e.g. streptomycin, gentamicin, cycloserine.

3. Antibiotics effective against both gram +ve and gram –ve bacteria and also rickettsiae and *Chlamydia* species, e.g. tetracyclines, chloramphenicol, amoxycillin, cephalosporins. According to spectrum of activity antibiotics are grouped as follows:
   a. *Narrow spectrum antibiotics:* The antibiotics which are selectively effective either on gram +ve bacteria or gram –ve bacteria or certain fungi or yeast are called narrow spectrum antibiotics, e.g. benzyl penicillin, erythromycin, vancomycin.
   b. *Broad spectrum antibiotics:* The antibiotics which are effective on a large number of pathogens, not only gram +ve and gram –ve bacteria but also affect the intracellular organisms like viruses and rickettsiae, chlamydia species, are called broad spectrum antibiotics, e.g. tetracyclines, chloramphenicol, streptomycin, amoxycillin.

A. PENICILLINS

Q 1. Who is the founder of penicillin? What is the source of penicillin? Give the classification, mechanism of action, adverse effects, therapeutic uses, dosage of penicillins.

Penicillins

Penicillin was discovered in 1929 by Alexander Fleming in England. It is extracted from the mould *Penicillium notatum* and *Penicillium chrysogenum.*

Classification

1. Natural penicillins, e.g. benzylpenicillin, phenoxymethyl penicillin.
2. Penicillinase resistant penicillins, e.g. cloxacillins, oxacillin, methicillin.
3. Broad spectrum penicillins, e.g. ampicillin, amoxycillin.
4. Penicillins active against Pseudomonas, e.g. carbenicillin.

Mechanism of Action

Penicillin is bactericidal in action. It is effective mainly against multiplying organisms.

Penicillins act by interfering with synthesis of bacterial cell wall. This makes the cell membrane of the organism possible to damage by soultes in the surrounding medium.

As the cell wall synthesis occurs during the growth phase, the antibiotic is most effective against actively multiplying organisms. The cell walls of gram –ve bacilli are chemically more complex. These cell walls contain β-lactamases in small amounts that are enough to inactivate penicillin.

Adverse Effects

i. Intolerance: It involves anaphylactic shock, idiosyncrasy and allergic reactions.

ii. Superinfection.
iii. Hyperkalemia: On administration of potassium salts of penicillins.
iv. Hypertension, palpitation, auditory and visual disturbance, headache.
v. Renal complications like haematuria, albuminuria.
vi. Thrombocytopenia, drug fever, eosinophilia, asthma, skin rash.

Test for Detection of Penicillin Allergy

A small quantity of penicillin solution containing 10,000 units/ml is injected intradermally.

If a central wheal due to local edema occurs after 15 minutes, it is considered as a positive reaction for penicillin allergy.

Therapeutic uses

i. To treat pneumococcal infections
ii. To treat streptococcal infections
iii. To treat staphylococcal infections
iv. To treat meningococcal infections
v. To treat syphilis and gonorrhoea
vi. To treat actinomycosis
vii. To treat anthrax
viii. To treat diphtheria, tetanus
ix. To treat rheumatic fever
x. To treat agranulocytosis

Preparation and Doses

Drug	*Brand name*	*Dose*	*Route*
1. Penicillin G potassium or sodium	Pentids Novapen	2–5 lakh units every 8 hours 3–8 million units/day	Tablets for oral use. Injection for IM, IV
2. Penicillin G benzathine	Penidure	Single dose of 6–12 lakh units every 1 or 2 weeks	IM injection
3. Penicillin G procaine	Crys – 4	6 lakh–1.2 million units every day	IM injection
4. Cloxacillin	Klox, Bioclox	250–1 gm four times a day	Oral (capsules)
5. Amoxycillin	Mox, Biomox Novamox	250–500 mg thrice a day	Oral (capsules)
6. Ampicillin	Ampillin, Rocillin	250–500 mg four times a day, half an hour before or 2 hours after meal	Oral, IM or IV
7. Ampicillin + cloxacillin	Ampilox, Amplus, Ampoxin, Biclopen	250–500 mg q.i.d.	Oral, IM or IV

B. CEPHALOSPORINS

Q 1. Write a note on 'cephalosporins'.

Cephalosporins

- Cephalosporins are a class of β-lactam antibodies originally derived from mold acremonium which was previously known as cephalosporum.
- Together with cephamycins, they constitute a subgroup of β-lactam antibiotics called cephems.
- Cephalosporins were discovered in 1945.

Classification

a. *First generation cephalosporins* (effective against gram-positive bacteria), e.g. cefazolin, cephalexin, cefadroxil.
b. *Second generation cephalosporins* (effective against gram-negative bacteria), e.g. cefuroxime, cefuroxime axetil, cefmetazole.
c. *Third generation cephalosporins:* They are less active than first generation, against gram-positive cocci but are strongly active against Enterobacteriaceae including β-lactamase producing strains, e.g. cefotaxime, ceftriaxone, cefpodoxime proxetil.
d. *Fourth generation cephalosporins:* They have extended spectrum of activity as compared to third generation, e.g. cefepine.

Examples of Cephalosporins

Ceftriaxone

It is a third generation cephalosporin antibiotic.

Uses/Indications

1. In septicemia
2. In pneumonia
3. In meningitis
4. In surgical prophylaxis for gonorrhoea

Adverse Effects

- Sores, ulcers
- Shortness of breath
- Chest pains
- Black, tarry stools
- Unusual tiredness or weakness

Contraindications

- Hypersensitivity
- Porphyria
- Hypoalbuminaemia

Dosage

Ceftriaxone injection.
Dose: 1 gm daily by IV

Brand Name

Rocephin.

C. AMINOGLYCOSIDES

Q 1. What are aminoglycoside antibiotics? Give examples. Write a short note on streptomycin.

Aminoglycoside Antibiotics

Aminoglycoside antibiotics are the amino sugars with glycosidic linkage.

They are highly effective against gram –ve bacteria, e.g. streptomycin, gentamicin, kanamycin, tobramycin, neomycin.

Streptomycin

It is obtained from *Streptomyces griseus.*

Mechanism of Action

- The ribosomes prepare enzymes under the directions from messengers RNA (mRNA).
- Streptomycin combines with bacterial ribosomes and interferes with mRNA ribosome combination and destroys the bacterial cell.
- According to another hypothesis streptomycin induces the ribosomes to manufacture peptide chains with wrong amino acids which ultimately destroy the bacterial cell.

Adverse Effects

1. *Ototoxicity:* Streptomycin causes damage to 8th cranial nerve (auditory nerve). Thus causes deafness.
2. *Nephrotoxicity:* Renal irritation, albuminuria.
3. *Superinfection:* Development of secondary infection during the course of primary infection.
4. *Intolerance:* Skin rash, eosinophilia, dermatitis, pericarditis.
5. Orally it may cause nausea, vomiting.

Therapeutic uses

Streptomycin is used in the treatment of:

1. Tuberculosis
2. Plague
3. Urinary tract infection
4. Meningitis due to *H. influenzae*
5. Bacteremia
6. Endocarditis
7. Respiratory tract infection
8. Gonorrhoea
9. Brucellosis.

Preparation

Streptomycin injection 0.5–200 mg intramuscularly per day.

D. FLUOROQUINOLONES

Q 1. What are fluoroquinolones? Explain nalidixic acid and ciprofloxacin.

Fluoroquinolones

- Fluoroquinolones are potent antibacterial agents.
- Quinolones are type of antibiotics.
- Fluoroquinolones are derived from quinolones by modifying their structure with fluorine.
- Examples of fluoroquinolones:
  1. Ciprofloxacin 2. Moxifloxacin 3. Gatifloxacin

1. Nalidixic Acid

- It is a urinary tract anti-infective agent (urinary antiseptic).
- It is a first synthetic quinolone antibiotic.
- The quinolones block DNA replication and repair by inhibiting DNA gyrase.
- Nalidixic acid is active against both gram-positive and gram-negative bacteria.

Adverse Effects

- Nausea, vomiting, diarrhoea
- Abdominal pain
- Dizziness, headache, drowsiness
- Insomnia, convulsions
- Rash, urticaria, photosensitivity, pruritus
- Blurred vision
- Depression, hallucinations
- Myalgia
- Hepatic dysfunction

Uses

1. In urinary tract infection (urinary antiseptic)
2. In shigellosis

Contraindications

- Hypersensitivity
- Pregnancy
- Convulsive disorder

Dosage

Nalidixic acid tab.

Dose: 1 gm every 6 hours for 7 days orally.

2. Ciprofloxacin

- Ciprofloxacin belongs to a class of drugs called quinolone antibiotics.

Uses/Indications

1. In urinary tract infections
2. In shigellosis
3. In travellers diarrhoea
4. In gastroenteritis
5. In respiratory tract infection
6. In cystic fibrosis
7. In bone and joint infection
8. In septicaemia
9. In skin infection

Adverse Effects

- Nausea, vomiting, diarrhoea
- Heartburn, stomach pains
- Pale skin
- Unusual tiredness

Dosage

Ciprofloxacin tablets.
Dose: 250–750 mg twice daily.

Brand Names

Cipro, CiproXR.

E. MACROLIDES

Q 1. What are macrolide antibiotics? Classify them with examples. Explain erythromycin and azithromycin.

Or

Write a note on 'macrolide antibiotics'.

Macrolide Antibiotics

- Macrolides are the class of natural products that consist of a large macrocyclic lactone ring to which one or more deoxy sugars are attached.
- Macrolide belongs to polyketide class of natural products.
- Macrolides are derived from *Saccharopolyspora erythraea.*
- Macrolide produces the action by binding to the 50S ribosomal subunit, thereby inhibiting the protein synthesis.

Classification

a. 1st generation macrolides, e.g. picromycin, erythromycin.
b. 2nd generation macrolides:
   i. 14-membered ring, e.g. clarithromycin, roxithromycin, flurithromycin, dirithromycin.
   ii. 15-membered ring, e.g. azithromycin.
c. 3rd generation macrolides, e.g. spiramycin, tylosin, carbomycin.

1. Erythromycin

It is a macrolide antibiotic.

Mechanism of Action

It inhibits protein synthesis at 50S ribosomal level.

Adverse Effects

1. Allergic reactions such as fever, eosinophilia, skin eruptions
2. Obstructive jaundice

3. Epigastric distress
4. Nausea, vomiting
5. Hepatitis

Therapeutic uses

1. In respiratory tract infections (whooping cough)
2. Sinusitis
3. Alternative to penicillin hypersensitive patients

Preparation

Erythromycin tablet 250–500 mg orally.
Trade name: Althrocin.

2. Azithromycin

It is more active than erythromycin against some gram-negative organisms.

Therapeutic uses

1. In uncomplicated genital chlamydial infections 2. In trachoma.

Adverse Effects

Anorexia, dyspepsia, constipation, dizziness, acute renal failure, hepatic necrosis.

Contraindications

Hepatic impairment.

Dosage

Azithromycin tablet.
Dose: 250–500 mg daily orally.

Brand Names

Azi, Azithral.

F. TETRACYCLINES

Q 1. Write a note on tetracycline antibiotics.

Tetracyclines

- Tetracyclines are broad spectrum antibiotics and are naphthalene derivatives.
- Chlortetracycline has been isolated from *Streptomyces aureofaciens* while oxytetracycline has been derived from *Streptomyces rimosus*.

Mechanism of Action

- Tetracyclines act by inhibiting certain enzyme system of the bacterial cell.
- They also suppress the synthesis of proteins in the microorganisms.

- Tetracyclines form complexes with certain cations like calcium and magnesium which are essential for the functional activity of various enzyme systems and ribosomes.
- Thus, tetracyclines are bacteriostatic in action.
- In higher concentrations or parenteral administration tetracyclines may exert a bactericidal effect.

Adverse Effects

1. On oral administration, it causes nausea, vomiting, epigastric distress, loose stools.
2. *Intolerance:* Pigmentation of teeth, a brown black colouration of teeth and nails, skin rash, dermatitis, blood dyscrasias.
3. *Superinfection:* Suppress of normal intestinal flora with resultant superinfection after prolonged tetracycline therapy.
4. *Liver toxicity:* Pancreatitis, fatty generation of liver, jaundice.
5. Toxicity on bones and teeth (defective bones and teeth)
   - Tetracycline chelates with calcium and, therefore, deposited in the areas of calcification in bones and teeth.
   - Administration of tetracycline to pregnant women may lead to yellow staining of the teeth of the infant, defective formation of enamel and hypoplasia of teeth may also occur.
   - Pigmentation of teeth and increased risk of caries may occur in children receiving a long- or short-term therapy of tetracyclines. Hence, tetracyclines should be avoided in infants and in children up to the age of 12 years.
   - Tetracyclines administered during pregnancy are deposited in foetal bones and may reduce a linear growth of the foetus. However, to prevent damage to the bones and teeth in the growing foetus, tetracyclines should be avoided after fourth month of pregnancy.
   - Tetracyclines are also deposited in the nails and fluorescence of nail may be demonstrated after prolonged tetracycline therapy.

Preparation

Tetracycline HCl capsule.

Dose: 1–3 gm daily in divided doses.

Trade Names

Tetracyn, Resteclin, Terramycin SF.

Therapeutic uses

1. In rickettsial infection
2. In plague
3. In cholera
4. In chlamydia infection
5. In bacillary infection
6. In urinary tract infection
7. In venereal diseases
8. In pneumonia
9. In respiratory tract infections.

Contraindications

1. Pregnancy
2. In children
3. Porphyria

QUESTIONS: GIVE THE REASONS

Q 1. Why penicillin is life-saving as well as life-threatening drug?

Penicillin is used in different diseases like:

i. Syphilis and gonorrhoea
ii. Diphtheria
iii. Gangrene
iv. Tetanux
v. Meningitis

Thus, it is life-saving drug.

Penicillin in therapeutic dose if randomly administered to an individual without checking its allergy then it may produce severe allergic reaction such as anaphylactic shock. Hence, it is life-threatening drug.

Q 2. Why antibiotics are generally given in combination?

i. The simultaneous use of two or more antibiotics has certain advantages and such combination is required in special situations. However, the effect of drug combination on the microorganisms as well as the host should be considered.
ii. The combined antibiotic therapy is indicated in the following conditions:
   a. Mixed bacterial infection, e.g. pulmonary or urogenital tract infection.
   b. Severe infection of unknown etiology, e.g. septic shock with UTI.
   c. To enhance antibacterial activity.

Hence, antibiotics are generally given in combination.

Q 3. Why penicillin kills many bacteria but spares host cells?

i. Penicillin is effectively mainly against multiplying organisms.
ii. It interferes with the synthesis of bacterial cell wall mucopeptide of gram-positive cocci.
iii. This makes the cell membrane of the organism susceptible to damage by solute in surrounding medium.
iv. A cell wall synthesis occurs during the growth phase. Thus, it acts as bactericidal.

v. It does not interfere with the tissue cell wall synthesis in human beings.
vi. Thus, it is non-toxic even in higher doses. Thus, it spares host cells.

Q 4. Why probenecid is sometimes given as an adjuvant in penicillin therapy?

i. Probenecid inhibits the renal tubular secretion of penicillin and thus increase or prolongs the blood level of penicillin.
ii. Probenecid does not have any direct antibacterial activity.
iii. Thus, for prolonging the blood levels of penicillin probenecid is administered along with penicillin.
iv. Another means of prolonging the serum levels of penicillin is the administration of repository preparation of penicillin G such as penicillin G procaine or penicillin G benzathine.

Q 5. Why are tetracyclines avoided to be given with milk or antacid?

i. Antacids contain Ca^{++}, Mg^{++}, Al^{+++} ions and milk contains Ca^{++} ions.
ii. Tetracyclines if administered with milk or antacid, form insoluble complexes with these ions.
iii. Due to formation of complexes, absorption of tetracycline is poor, inadequate thus reduces pharmacological action of tetracycline.

Hence, tetracyclines are avoided to be given with milk or antacids.

Q 6. Why are tetracyclines called broad spectrum antibiotics?

i. The tetracyclines are effective against large number of pathogens not only gram-positive and gram-negative bacteria but also affect the intracellular organisms like viruses, rickettsiae, chlamydia, actinomyces.
ii. As the tetracyclines have a wide spectrum or activity hence they are called broad spectrum antibiotics.

Q 7. Why tetracyclines are contraindicated/avoided in pregnant women and children?

i. Administration of tetracycline during pregnancy, cause deposition of tetracycline in foetal bones and may reduce the growth of foetus.
ii. Tetracyclines are also deposited in growing teeth and bones and if treatment is very prolonged the nail become stained by stored tetracycline.
iii. Children may show brown staining of teeth if tetracyclines are administered before the appearance of first tooth. Pigmentation of permanent teeth may take place.
iv. Thus, damage to both deciduous and permanent teeth occurs.
v. Deposition of tetracyclines in the growing ends of bones can cause stunted growth.

Hence, tetracycline is contraindicated in pregnant women and children.

Objective Questions with Answers in Bold Letters

1. The agents which stop the growth of bacteria are called **bacteriostatic**.
2. **Bacteriocides** are the agents which kill the bacteria.
3. **Alexander flexing** is a founder of penicillin.
4. Oxacillin is a **penicillinase resistant penicillin.**
5. Penicillin is effective against **multiplying** organisms.
6. **Anaphylactic shock** is a major toxic effect of penicillins.
7. Penicillin acts by **interfering with synthesis of bacterial cell wall.**
8. Cephalosporins are **β-lactam antibiotics.**
9. Cephalosporin are originally derived from mold **acremonium.**
10. Cephalosporin antibiotic was discovered in **1945**.
11. **Streptomycin and gentamicin** are aminoglycoside antibiotics.
12. Streptomycin is obtained from ***Streptomyces griseus***.
13. **Ototoxicity** is a major drawback of streptomycin.
14. Streptomycin is used in the treatment of **tuberculosis**.
15. Ciprofloxacin is a **fluoroquinolone derivative.**
16. **Nalidixic acid** is used in urinary tract infection.
17. Ciprofloxacin is used in treatment of **"travellers diarrhoea."**
18. Erythromycin and azithromycin are **macrolide antibiotics**.
19. Macrolides are produced from ***Saccharopolyspora erythraea***.
20. Erythromycin inhibits protein synthesis at **50S ribosomal level**.
21. Tetracyclines are **naphthalene** derivatives.
22. Chlortetracycline has been isolated from ***Streptomyces aurefaciens***.
23. Oxytetracycline has been derived from ***Streptomyces rimosus***.
24. Tetracycline acts by **inhibiting enzyme system** of bacterial cell.
25. **Pigmentation of teeth** is a toxicity of tetracycline.
26. **Tetracyclines** are contraindicated in pregnant women and children.
27. Tetracycline is a drug of choice in treatment of plague.
28. **Penicillin** is a life-saving as well as life-threatening drug.
29. **Probenecid** is given as an adjuvant in penicillin therapy.
30. **Tetracyclines** should be avoided with milk or antacid.

G. SULPHONAMIDES

Q 1. What are sulphonamides? Classify sulphonamides giving examples. Explain mechanism of action of sulphonamides.

Sulphonamides

Definition

The antimicrobial compounds containing sulphonamide group ($-SO_2NH_2$) are called sulphonamides.

Classification

1. For systemic use:
   a. Short-acting sulphonamides, e.g. sulphadiazine, sulphacetamide, sulphadimidine.
   b. Intermediate-acting sulphonamides, e.g. sulphamethoxazole.
   c. Long-acting sulphonamides, e.g. sulphamethoxypyridazine.
2. For GIT infection, e.g. sulphaguanidine, succinyl sulphathiazole, sulphasalazine, pthalylsulphathiazole.

Mechanism of Action

i. Sulphonamide has structural similarity to p-aminobenzoic acid (PABA).
ii. Hence, it competes with PABA in bacterial metabolism.
iii. Folic acid derived from PABA is important in bacterial metabolism.
iv. Sulphonamide inhibits the enzyme folic acid synthetase which is useful for conversion of PABA into folic acid.
v. This causes folic acid deficiency resulting in injury to the bacterial cell.
vi. Such injured cells can be phagocytosed easily.

PABA
↓
Folic acid
↓
Dihydrofolic acid
↓
Tetrahydrofolic acid (folinic acid)
↓
Purine (DNA) synthesis
↓
Bacterial growth

Q 2. Give the adverse effects and therapeutic uses of sulphonamides/sulpha drugs.

Adverse Effects (Toxic Effects) of Sulphonamides

i. *Intolerance:* Skin rash, toxic hepatitis, toxic nephritis, acute haemolytic anemia.

ii. *Urinary toxicity:* Renal irritation, obstruction in urine flow, haematuria, albuminuria, crystalluria.
iii. *Haemopoietic system:* Aplastic anemia, agranulocytosis, intravascular hemolysis.

Therapeutic uses of Sulphonamides

i. In urinary tract infections
ii. In acute bacillary dysentery
iii. In GIT infection
iv. In influenza
v. In meningitis
vi. In meningococcal meningitis
vii. In conjunctivitis
viii. In rheumatoid arthritis.

Q 3. What is cotrimoxazole? Give its mechanism of action, uses, adverse effects, dosage and brand names.

Cotrimoxazole

- Cotrimoxazole is a mixture of 5 parts of sulphamethoxazole and 1 part of trimethoprim.
- These two components of co-trimoxazole interferes with the bacterial synthesis of tetrahydrofolic acid which is an essential stage in the production of nucleic acid.

Adverse Effects

- Nausea, vomiting, headache
- Rash, urticaria
- Hepatitis
- Agranulocytosis
- Renal colic
- Mental depression

Contraindications

- Hypersensitivity to sulphonamides
- Pregnancy
- Lactation
- Liver disease
- Renal impairment

Uses

It is used in:
- Urinary tract infections.
- Respiratory tract infections like bronchitis, pneumonia.
- Meningitis.
- Enteric infections like typhoid and paratyphoid.
- Ear infections such as otitis media.

Mechanism of Action

- PABA is essential for bacterial growth.
- Sulphamethoxazole and trimethoprim act synergistically by blocking the formation of folic acid and its utilisation. This combination is called co-trimoxazole (5:1).

- Sulphamethoxazole inhibits the conversion of PABA into dihydrofolic acid by inhibiting the enzyme dihydrofolic acid synthetase.
- Trimethoprim inhibits conversion of dihydrofolic acid into tetrahydrofolic acid by inhibiting the enzyme dihydrofolic acid reductase.
- Tetrahydrofolic acid (THFA) is necessary in pruine and DNA synthesis.
- So, cotrimoxazole inhibits both steps in bacterial metabolism and acts as antibacterial.

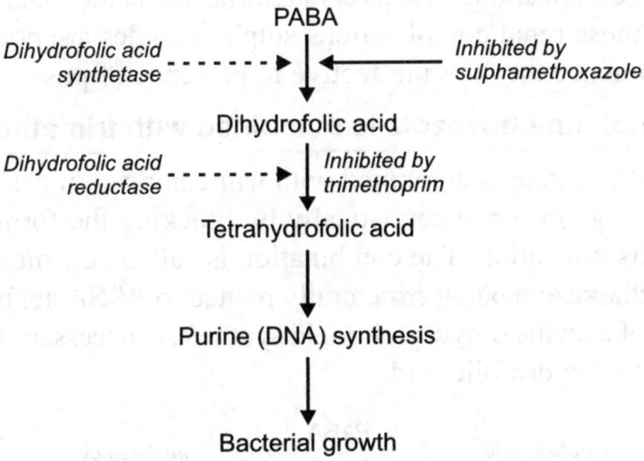

QUESTIONS: GIVE THE REASONS

Q 1. Why large amount of fluid and alkali is given with sulfa drugs?

Or

Why patient on sulfa therapy is advised to drink more water?

Or

Why simultaneously antacid therapy is given to patient on sulfa drugs?

i. Sulphonamides cause renal complications.
ii. In presence of acidic urine the acetylated form of sulphonamide is precipitated in collecting tubules and calyces.
iii. This causes renal irritation, obstruction of urinary flow, crystalluria, albuminuria, haematuria, oliguria and anuria.
iv. The acetylated form of sulphonamide is soluble in alkaline urine.
v. Alkalinisation of urine also enhances the urinary excretion of sulphonamides.
vi. Hence, large amount of fluid or alkalis or simultaneous antacid therapy is given to make the urine alkaline and to minimise chances of renal complications.

Q 2. Why sulphonamides are not effective in presence of pus?

i. PABA (p-aminobenzoic acid) is required for synthesis of folic acid.
ii. Due to structural similarity with sulphonamide it is competitive inhibitor of PABA.
iii. Since, pus contains large amount of PABA, sulphonamides in therapeutic dose are not effective.
iv. If the larger dose of sulphonamide is used to complete with PABA, it results into renal complications such as crystalluria, haematuria and renal damage.
v. To avoid these renal complications sulphonamides are not used in large doses and hence they are ineffective in presence of pus.

Q 3. Why sulphamethoxazole is combined with trimethoprim?

i. Sulphamethoxazole is combined with trimethoprim in 5:1 ratio.
ii. These two agents act synergistically by blocking the formation of folic acid and its utilisation. The combination is called cotrimoxazole.
iii. Sulphamethoxazole being structurally related to PABA act by competitive blockade of enzyme dihydrofolic acid synthetase, necessary for conversion of PABA to dihydrofolic acid.

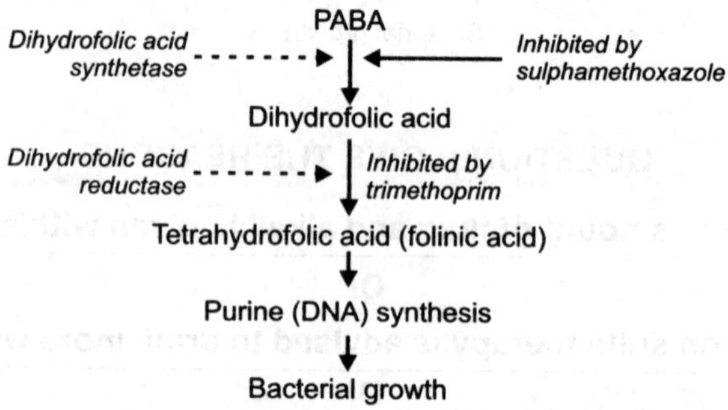

iv. Trimethoprim interferes with the action of dihydrofolic acid reductase.
v. This enzyme is necessary for conversion of dihydrofolic acid to tetrahydrofolic acid, which is an essential stage in the bacterial purine and DNA synthesis.
vi. Thus, the sequential blockade produced by these two drugs explains the synergistic effect.
vii. In combination of these two drugs also overcomes each other's side effects.

Q 4. Why phthalyl sulphathiazole and succinyl sulphathiazole are not effective *in vitro*?

i. These are the prodrugs used in the treatment of bacillary dysentery and to sterilise the intestinal tract prior to surgery. These are poorly absorbed compounds.

ii. The phthalyl or succinyl radical is attached to the p-amino group.
iii. In the colon the microbial flora split the drug to release sulphathiazole which is the active part.

Hence, these two drugs are not effective *in vitro* (outside the body).

H. ANTITUBERCULAR AGENTS

Q 1. What is tuberculosis? Define and classify antitubercular agents with suitable examples.

Or

Write a note on antitubercular agents.

Tuberculosis

Tuberculosis is a disease caused by an organism *Mycobacterium tuberculosis.*

1. Antitubercular Agents

The drugs which are used in the treatment of tuberculosis are called antitubercular drugs.

Classification

1. **Standard drugs/primary drugs/first line drugs**, e.g. isoniazid (INH), rifampicin (R), ethambutol (E), streptomycin (S), pyrazinamide (Z), p-aminosalicylic acid (PAS), thiacetazone.
2. **Reserve drugs/secondary drugs/second line drugs**, e.g. kanamycin (K), capreomycin (Cm), cycloserine (C).

2. Isoniazid (Isonicotinic Acid Hydrazide) (INH)

It is most effective and cheapest antitubercular agent.

Mechanism of Action

Isoniazid inhibits the enzymes essential for synthesis of mycobacterial cell walls.

Isoniazid inhibits phospholipid synthesis and damages the membrane of tubercle bacilli. Intracellular and extracellular chelation of divalent cations essential for bacterial metabolism is another possible mechanism of action.

INH suppresses the formation of DNA and RNA and also inhibits various oxidative mechanisms.

Adverse Effects

1. Peripheral neuritis, hepatotoxicity, anaemia.
2. Convulsions, loss of memory, loss of self-control.

Preparation of Antitubercular Drugs

1. Isoniazid tablet IP	: 200–300 mg daily in a single dose	: Isokin, : Isonex
2. Rifampicin tablet IP	: 10 mg/kg daily	: Rifamycin

Q 2. Give the reason. "In tuberculosis treatment drug combination is preferred than single drug treatment". Why?

Or

In tuberculosis, the drugs are given synergistically.

The combination drug therapy in treatment of tuberculosis is preferred because of its following advantages over the single drug therapy:

i. Resistance to antitubercular drug is developed fastly if used single than combination treatment.
ii. Combination therapy avoids the viability and multiplication of bacilli during treatment.
iii. Combined drug therapy gives the synergistic effect.
iv. It avoids caseation which tends to block the blood vessels supplying to necrotic area and making penetration by antitubercular drug difficult.

I. ANTIFUNGAL DRUGS

Q 1. Enlist various fungal infections. Define and classify antifungal agents giving suitable examples.

Fungal Infections

- Any disease caused by fungus is known as fungal infection.
- Fungi are heterotropic microorganisms.
- A fungal infection is also called mycosis, a skin disease caused by a fungus.
- Mycotic infections of human are:
  1. Dermatophytosis is a contagious superficial skin infection. The diseases produced are ringworm of foot, ringwarm of skin, hair, nails.
  2. Candidiasis can affect the skin and mucus membrane.
  3. Saprophytes invade skin and penetrate deep causing lymphatic, pulmonary and systemic mycoses.

Fungal infections are:

i. Candidiasis: Caused by yeast Candida.
ii. Blastomycosis: Caused by the fungus Blastomyces.
iii. Ringworm: A common fungal infection.
iv. Vaginal candidiasis.
v. Fungal nail infections.
vi. Mucormycosis: Caused by mucormycetes.
vii. Onchomycosis.
viii. Histoplasmosis.

Antifungal Agents

The drugs which are used in the treatment of fungal infections are called antifungal agents.

Classification

1. ***Antifungal antibiotics:***
   a. Polyene macrolide, e.g. amphotericin, nystatin.
   b. Non-polyene, e.g. griseofulvin.
2. ***Synthetic:***
   a. Imidazole derivatives, e.g. ketoconazole, miconazole, clotrimazole.
   b. Triazole derivatives, e.g. fluconazole, itraconazole.
3. ***Unsaturated fatty acid:*** Undecylenic acid.
4. ***Thiocarbanilic acid derivative:*** Tolnaftate.

Q 2. Write a note on any four antifungal drugs.

Antifungal Drugs

1. Griseofulvin

Griseofulvin is an antibiotic isolated from *Penicillium griseofulvum* and is selectively effective in dermatophyte infections of the skin, nails and hair.

Mechanism of Action

It inhibits fungal mitosis by interfering with microtubule function.

Therapeutic uses

1. As an antifungal agent.
2. To treat fungal infections of skin, scalp, hair and nail.
3. Used to treat dermatophytoses.
4. Used to treat ringworm infection.
5. Used to treat tinea infections.
6. Effective in aspergillus and candida infections.

Adverse Effects

- Nausea, vomiting
- Flushing
- Peripheral neuritis
- Mental confusion, fatigue

Contraindications

- Severe liver disease
- Porphyria

Dosage

Griseofulvin tablets.

Dose: 500 mg daily in single or divided dose orally.

Brand Names

G-fulvin, Grisovin-FP.

2. Nystatin

- Nystatin is a polylene macrolide antibiotic.
- It was isolated from *Streptomyces noursei* and is very effective in the treatment of yeast infections such as candida.

Therapeutic uses/Indications

1. To prevent or treat superficial candidiasis of mouth, oesophagus, intestinal tract.
2. To treat vaginal candidiasis.
3. As a fungistatic and fungicidal.
4. In *Blastomyces dermatitidis*.

Adverse Effects

- Nausea, vomiting, diarrhoea
- Stomach pain or upset
- Stevens-Johnson syndrome
- Hypersensitivity reactions
- Skin irritation or redness

Dosage

Nystatin tablets.

Dose: 5 lakh units every 6 hours.

Brand Names

Nystan, Nystaform, Nystaderm.

3. Amphotericin B

- It is a natural polyene macrolide.
- It is produced by *Streptomyces nodosus* and used for the treatment of yeast infections.
- It is a complimentary antifungal drug.

Uses/Indications

1. In candidiasis, blastomycosis
2. In cryptococcal meningitis
3. In mucormycosis
4. In histoplasmosis
5. In coccidioidomycosis
6. For the suppression of oral or intestinal candidiasis.

Adverse Effects

- Fever, chills
- Vomiting, headache
- Muscle spasms
- Hypotension
- Renal toxicity

Dosage

Amphotericin B tablet.

Dose: 200 mg every 6 hours orally.

Brand Names

Fungizone, Fungilin.

4. Fluconazole

- It is a triazole derivative.
- It is a representative azole antifungal.

Uses/Indications

1. In histoplasmosis
2. In non-meningeal coccidioidomycosis
3. In blastomycosis
4. In oesophageal and oropharyngeal candidiasis
5. In vaginal and systemic candidiasis.

Adverse Effects

- Chest tightness
- Difficulty in swallowing
- Skin rash or itching
- Light coloured stools
- Stomach pain

Dosage

Fluconazole tablet.

Dose: 200 mg daily orally.

Brand Names

Diflucan, Fluka.

J. ANTIVIRAL DRUGS

Q 1. Give an account of antiviral drugs.

Antiviral Drugs

The drugs which are used in the treatment of viral infections are called antiviral drugs.

Examples of antiviral drugs:

1. Idoxuridine
2. Amantidine
3. Zidovudine
4. Ribavirin
5. Nelfinavir
6. Acyclovir
7. Favipiravir
8. Remdesivir
9. Thiosemicarbazones
10. Interferons
11. Human immunoglobulins
12. Ritonavir

Classification

1. Drugs acting as antiherpesvirus, e.g. idoxuridine, acyclovir, favipiravir, foscarnet.
2. Drugs acting as anti-influenza virus, e.g. amantadine.
3. Drugs acting as antihepatitis virus, e.g. ribavirin.
4. Drugs acting as antiretrovirus, e.g. zidovudine.

1. Idoxuridine (IDU, IUDR)

- It is a first antiviral drug approved.
- It is a substituted pyrimidine analogue.
- It is used topically in the treatment of herpes keratitis (0.1% solution).

Therapeutic uses

1. It is an antiviral agent against herpesvirus.
2. It is used for topical treatment of herpes keratitis.
3. It is used for the treatment of herpes labialis, genitalis, and zoster.
4. It is used for the topical treatment of herpes simplex virus (HSV) keratitis.
5. It is used in ophthalmic for the treatment of HSV keratoconjunctivitis.

Adverse Effects

- Rendess, itching
- Eye irritation or pain
- Swelling of eye
- Increased sensitivity to light and glare

Dosage

Idoxuridine ophthalmic solutions : 1%.
Idoxuridine ophthalmic ointment : 0.5%.

Brand Names

Herplex, Idrin, Xurin.

2. Amantadine

- It is a synthetic tricyclic amine which prevents replication of influenza virus.
- This substance inhibits some myxoviruses such as human influenza and parainfluenza.

Therapeutic uses

1. It is used as an antiviral drug.
2. It is used in the treatment of various strains of influenza A virus.

3. Amantadine is used in the treatment of Parkinson's disease.
4. It is also used as a dopamine receptor agonist.
5. Amantadine is used for the treatment of many prototypes of influenza A virus (H_1N_1, H_2N_2, Asian type, H_3N_2).
6. Amantadine is used for the treatment of cerebral arteriosclerosis.
7. It is used to releive fatigue.

Adverse Effects

- Dryness of mouth
- Nausea, vomiting, headache
- Constipation
- Loss of appetite
- Abnormal dreams

Dosage

Amantadine tablets/capsules.

Dose: 100–200 gm daily in two dividied doses, orally.

Brand Names

Amantral, Comantrel, Neaman.

3. Interferons

- Interferons are low molecular weight glycoproteins produced by host cells in response to a viral infection.
- The antiviral action of interferons is very broad and they are effective against a wide range of unrelated viruses.
- Interferons are effective in a wide variety of RNA and DNA of viruses and viral multiplication is stopped.

Adverse Effects

- Headache, fever
- Depression
- Lethargy
- Dizziness

Dosage

Interferon is available as injections containing recombinant human interferon 2B, 3 million IU injection and 5 million IU per vial.

4. Human Immunoglobulins

- The normal human plasma contains antibodies to protect from many diseases.
- The antibodies are in gammaglobulin.
- Human immunoglobulins have five classes IgA, IgD, IgE, IgG and IgM which are present in serum and secretions of the body.

5. Immunological Methods

The use of prophylactic vaccination is one of the best ways for prevention of viral infections.

6. Acyclovir

- Acyclovir is an antiviral drug.
- It is effective against herpes simplex viruses type 1 and type 2, varicella-zoster virus and other viruses of the herpesvirus family.

Mechanism of Action

It acts by interfering with DNA synthesis by conversion to acyclovir trisulphate which causes decrease in viral replication.

Therapeutic uses

1. In herpes simplex
2. In herpes genitalis
3. In herpes zoster
4. In chickenpox

Adverse Effects

- Tremors, headache, nausea, vomiting
- Lethargy
- Abdominal pains, colitis
- Hematuria, vaginitis
- Skin rash, urticaria
- Joint pains, muscle cramps
- Acute renal failure

Dosage

Acyclovir tablet IP.

Dose: 200–800 mg, 4–5 times daily orally.

Brand Names

Acivir, Herpex-200, Cyclovir.

7. Remdesivir

- Remdesivir is a prodrug of an adenosine triphosphate (ATP) analogue.
- Remdesivir has potential antiviral activity against a variety of RNA viruses.
- Remdesivir is first described in the literature in 2016 as a potential treatment of Ebola.
- Remdesivir being a prodrug, is metabolized into its active form GS-441524.

Adverse Effects

- Back pain
- Chest tightness
- Flushing
- Headache
- Itching
- Nausea, vomiting
- Swelling of the eyelids
- Dark coloured stools

Therapeutic uses

1. Remdesivir is used for the treatment of coronavirus disease 2019 (COVID-19) infection requiring hospitalization.
2. It is useful for the treatment of SARS-COV-2 virus in hospitalized adult and children 12 years of age.

3. Remdesivir is an antiviral drug.
4. Remdesivir helps to stop the spread of the virus throughout the body.
5. Remdesivir is used as a potential treatment of Ebola.
6. Remdesivir activity against the Coronaviridae family was first demonstrated in 2017, for the treatment of COVID-19.

Pharmaceutical Formulations

1. Remdesivir injection.
2. Remdesivir lyophilized powder for reconstitution.

Brand Names

Covifor, Veklury, Redyx, Cipremi, Remdac.

Dose: By IV 200 mg as a single dose on day 1, followed by 100 mg once daily. Duration is generally 5 days.

8. Favipiravir

- Favipiravir is a pyrazine carboxamide derivative with activity against RNA viruses.
- It is an antiviral drug used to manage influenza that has the potential to target other viral infections.
- Favipiravir is known to be teratogenic, therefore, should be avoided in pregnancy conditions.
- Favipiravir is extensively metabolized with metabolites exerted mainly in the urine.

Adverse Effects

- Hyperuricemia
- Diarrhoea
- Reduced neutrophil count
- Nausea, vomiting
- Abdominal pains

Therapeutic uses

1. Favipiravir is an antiviral drug used to manage influenza.
2. Used in the treatment of avian influenza.
3. Recently favipiravir is used in COVID-19 infection and has the potential to target other viral infections.

Pharmaceutical Formulation

Favipiravir tablet.

Brand Names

Avifavir, Areplivir, Avigan, Favimed, BAL Flu.

Dose: 1800 mg orally twice daily for COVID-19.

Q 2. Give a brief account of "drug used in HIV infection."

Drugs used in HIV Infection

- Human immunodeficiency virus (HIV) infection cannot be cured by antiretroviral drugs but only can be suppressed to improve the symptoms.
- Antiviral drugs are synthetic agents that have antiviral activity against HIV and are used in the management of HIV infection.
- They are four different classes of antiretroviral agents commercially available:
  1. Nucleoside reverse transcriptase inhibitors (NRTI), e.g. zidovudine, lamivudine, tavudine.
  2. Protease inhibitors, e.g. ritonavir, indinavir, saquinavir.
  3. Non-nucleoside reverse transcriptase inhibitors (NNRT), e.g. delavirdine (DLV), nevirapine.
  4. Fusion inhibitors, e.g. enfluvirtide (T_{20}).

1. Lamivudine

- Lamivudine is a nucleoside reverse transcriptase inhibitor.
- Lamivudine (3TC) is a nucleoside analog with *in vitro* activity against HIV-1, including zidovudine resistant strains and HBV.
- Lamivudine inhibits the reverse transcriptase of HIV-1 and is synergistic with zidovudine against HIV-1.
- Lamivudine, administered in combination with zidovudine or another nucleoside analogue retard the emergence of resistance, is indicated for the treatment of advance HIV disease.

Uses/Indications

In HIV infection in combination with at least two other antiviral drugs.

Adverse Effects

- Headache
- Insomnia
- Fatigue
- GIT discomfort
- Life-threatening lactic acidosis
- Thrombocytopenia
- Red cell aplasia

Dosage

Lamivudine tablets 150 mg.

Dose: 150 mg twice daily or 300 mg once daily orally.

Brand Names

Epivir, Epivir-HBV.

2. Zidovudine (Azidothymidine)

- Zidovudine is a nucleoside reverse transcriptase inhibitor.
- Zidovudine (AZT) is a deoxythymidine analogue.
- Zidovudine has *in vitro* activity against HIV-1, HIV-2 and the human T cell lympotropic viruses.

Therapeutic uses

1. Useful in HIV-1 infected individuals.
2. As a monotherapy for prevention of maternal-fetal HIV transmission.
3. Zidovudine has efficacy in the treatment of HIV-associated encephalopathy and thrombocytopenia.
4. Used in prevention of vertical transmission of HIV.

Adverse Effects

- Headache, insomnia
- Myelosuppression
- Gastrointestinal intolerance
- Thrombocytopenia
- Acute cholestatic hepatitis
- Myopathy

Dosage

Zidovudine tablet, capsule.

Dose: 500–600 mg daily in divided doses orally.

Brand Names

AZT, Retrovir, Ziddivir.

Protease Inhibitors

Drug	*Brand name*	*Dose*	*Route*
1. Ritonavir	Norvir	100 mg twice daily	Oral
2. Nelfinavir	Viracept	1.25 gm twice daily	Oral

Objective Questions with Answers in Bold Letters

1. The causative agent of tuberculosis is **bacterium.**
2. Nephrotoxicity is a common adverse effect of **amphotericin B**.
3. Acyclovir inhibits **herpesviruses.**
4. Tuberculosis is caused by ***Mycobacterium tuberculosis***.
5. PABA stands for **para-aminobenzoic acid**.
6. INH stands for **isonicotinic acid hydrazide**.
7. PAS stands for **para-aminosalicylic acid.**
8. **Sulphaguanidine** is effective in GIT infections.
9. Sulphacetamide is indicated for the treatment of **eye infections**.
10. **Sulphonamides** have a structural similarity to PABA.

11. **Crystalluria** is a major toxicity of sulphonamides.
12. Cotrimoxazole is a combination of **5 parts of sulphamethoxazole and 1 part of trimethoprim.**
13. PABA is essential for **purine (DNA) synthesis/bacterial growth.**
14. THF stands for **tetrahydrofolic acid.**
15. Large amount of fluid/alkali is given with **sulpha drugs.**
16. Sulphamethoxazole and trimethoprim is combined in the ratio of **5:1.**
17. **Peripheral neuritis** is a toxicity of isoniazid.
18. In tuberculosis treatment drugs are given **synergistically.**
19. Undecylenic acid is an **antifungal drug.**
20. Nystatin is a polyene **macrolide** antibiotic.
21. Stevens-Johnson syndrome is an adverse effect of **nystatin.**
22. **Fungizone** is a popular brand name of amphotericin B.
23. **Fluconazole** is used in the treatment of candidiasis and histoplasmosis.
24. **Idoxuridine** is an antiviral drug.
25. **Acyclovir** is an antiviral drug used in treatment of herpes simplex.
26. Remdesivir is a prodrug of an **adenosine triphosphate (ATP)** analogue.
27. Remdesivir being a prodrug, is metabolized into its active form **GS-441524.**
28. Remdesivir activity against the Coronaviridae family was first demonstrated in 2017, for the treatment of **COVID-19.**
29. Zidovudine and lamivudine are antiviral drugs used in the treatment of **HIV infections.**
30. Zidovudine is a **nucleoside reverse transcriptase inhibitor.**
31. Ritonavir and nelfinavir are **protease inhibitors** which are used in HIV infection.

K. ANTIAMOEBIC DRUGS

Q 1. What is amoebiasis? Define and classify antiamoebic agents.

Amoebiasis

It is an acute or chronic infection caused by the protozoan *Entamoeba histolytica.*

Antiamoebic Agents

The drugs which are used in the treatment of amoebic infection are called antiamoebic drugs.

Classification

- Natural alkaloid, e.g. emetine.
- Synthetic:
  i. Quinoline derivative, e.g. iodoquinol, clioquinol, iodohydroxyquin.
  ii. Imidazole derivative, e.g. metronidazole.

iii. Furan derivative, e.g. diloxanide furoate.
iv. Organometallic compound, e.g. acetarsol.
v. Dyes, e.g. gentian violet.

Q 2. Describe the drugs used in amoebiasis (antiamoebic drugs).

1. Emetine Hydrochloride

- It is an alkaloid isolated from ipecacuahna and is quickly effective in the suppression of acute amoebic dysentery.
- Emetine is administered parenterally.

Therapeutic uses

1. In amoebic dysentery.
2. In intestinal and hepatic amoebiasis.
3. In amoebic infection of lungs, brain and other tissues.

Adverse Effects

- Pain, tenderness, muscle weakness
- Hypotension
- Localised peripheral neuritis

Dosage

Emetine hydrochloride injection.

Dose: 65 mg daily for 5 days by SC or IM injection.

Brand Names

Dehydroemetine, Tilemetin.

2. Diloxanide Furoate

- It is an amoebicidal agent given orally.
- It is active against amoeba in the bowel lumen and inchronic cyst-passing states to give about 90% cure rate.

Uses

1. In the treatment of amoebic dysentery.
2. In hepatic amoebiasis.

Adverse Effects

- Flatulence
- Nausea, diarrhoea
- Abdominal cramps

Dosage

Diloxanide furoate tablets.

Dose: 500 mg every 8 hours for 10 days.

Brand Names

Diloxyl, Entamizole, Furamide.

3. Metronidazole

It is the drug of choice in most forms of amoebiasis.

On oral administration, it is completely absorbed from small intestine.

Adverse Effects

1. Metallic taste in mouth
2. Nausea, vomiting, headache
3. Abdominal pain
4. Stomatitis
5. Neurotoxicity
6. Allergic reactions—urticaria, pruritus

Therapeutic uses

1. In amoebiasis
2. In trichomoniasis
3. In giardiasis
4. In ulcerative stomatitis
5. In trichomonal vaginitis

Contraindications

- Alcoholism
- Seizures
- Peripheral neuropathy

Dosage

Metronidazole tablets IP.

Dose: 600–800 mg thrice daily, orally.

Brand Names

Metrogyl, Flagyl, Metroquin.

4. Arsenicals

The organic arsenic compounds have been used in the treatment of intestinal amoebiasis.

For example: Carbarsone, glycobiarsol.

5. Iodinated 8-hydroxyquinolones

These drugs such as chiniofon, diiodohydroxyquin and clioquinol may be used in intestinal amoebiasis. Clinoquinol has a popular reputation as a prophylactic and treatment of mild infective enteritis.

L. ANTHELMINTICS (ANTIWORMS)

Q 1. What are anthelmintics? Explain anthelmintic drugs.

Anthelmintics

The drugs which are used in the treatment of worm infestations are called anthelmintics, e.g. mebendazole, albendazole, thiabendazole, pyrantel pamoate, niclosamide, piperazine, DEC.

- **Vermicidal or wormicidal:** The drugs which kill or destroy the worms are called vermicidal or wormicidal agents.

- **Vermifuge or wormifuge:** The drugs which act on the worms in such a way that they can be easily expelled out, are known as vermifuges.
- **Requirement of an ideal anthelmintic:**
  1. It should have a broad spectrum action.
  2. It should achieve a high percentage of cure with a single dose.
  3. The purgation before and following the anthelmintic should not be necessary.
  4. It should not get absorbed.
  5. It should be palatable and cheap.
  6. It should be free from toxic effects.

Anthelmintic Drugs

1. **Piperazine**
   - It can be used against infestation with roundworms.
   - It is most widely used for ascariatic therapy.
2. **Mebendazole**
   - It is a broad spectrum anthelmintic.
   - It is used to treat roundworm, tapeworm, threadworm, hookworm, guineaworm infestation.
3. **Pyrantel pamoate:** It is effective in ascariasis and oxyguriasis.
4. **Diethylcarbamazine (DEC)**
   - It is used to treat anchocerciasis and filariasis.
   - To treat roundworm infestation and topical esosinophilia.
5. **Tetramisole:** It is used in the treatment of ascariasis.
6. **Albendazole:** It is a broad spectrum anthelmintic.

Anthelmintic Drugs (Preparation and Doses)

Drug	*Brand name*	*Dose*	*Route*
1. Mebendazole	Mebex, Wormin	100 mg twice daily for 3 days	Oral
2. Albendazole	Albex, Zentel	400 mg single dose with meals	Oral
3. Piperazine	Antepar	3.5 gm once daily for 2 days	Oral
4. Pyrantel pamoate	Nemocid	1 gm daily	Oral
5. Tetramisole	Jetomisol-P	150 mg daily	Oral
6. Diethylcarbamazine	Filazine, Banocide Forte	50 mg daily	Oral

Q 2. Why use of purgatives is essential with piperazine?

Or

Why anthelmintics are administered with purgatives?

- Anthelmintics are either wormicidal or wormifugal in action.
- Thus, after killing or paralysing these worms by anthelmintic agent, these should be expelled out from the intestine.
- Hence, purgatives are advised as supportive treatment with anthelmintics.
- Thus, combination acts synergistically.

M. ANTIMALARIAL DRUGS

Q 1. What is malaria? Give its causative agents. Define and classify antimalarial drugs.

Malaria

It is caused by parasitic protozoa of the genus Plasmodium which includes four types:

- *Plasmodium vivax*
- *Plasmodium falciparum*
- *Plasmodium ovale*
- *Plasmodium malariae*

1. Antimalarials

The drugs which are used in the treatment of malaria are called antimalarials.

Classification

1. Cinchona alkaloids, e.g. quinine
2. 4-aminoquinolines, e.g. chloroquine, amodiaquine
3. 8-aminoquinolines, e.g. primaquine
4. Acridine, e.g. mepacrine
5. Biguanides, e.g. proguanil
6. Diaminopyrimidines, e.g. pyrimethamine
7. Quinoline methanol, e.g. mefloquine
8. Miscellaneous, e.g. sulphonamides, tetracyclines.

Q 2. Write a note on the following antimalarial agents: (1) Quinine, (2) Chloroquine.

1. Quinine

It is an alkaloid obtained from cinchona bark.

Mechanism of Action

Quinine is schizonticidal and, therefore, useful as a suppressive.

Quinine has been termed a general protoplasmic poison. It depresses the variety of enzymatic processes and reduces ciliary activity and inhibits phagocytosis and growth of fibroblasts.

Adverse Effects

1. Cinchonism
2. Black water fever
3. Nephrotoxicity
4. Ringing in ears
5. Blurring of vision
6. Nausea, vomiting
7. Disturbances of colour vision
8. Acute renal damage
9. Ventricular arrhythmia
10. Deafness

Therapeutic uses

i. In malaria
ii. In cramps

Preparation

Quinine hydrochloride tablet IP.

Dose: 300–600 mg daily.

Brand Names

Vigo-tablet, Fluo-foe.

2. Chloroquine

It is a drug of choice in malaria.

Chloroquine is superior to quinine and mepacrine.

Mechanism of Action

Chloroquine acts by inhibiting the incorporation of phosphate into RNA and DNA of plasmodia.

Adverse Reactions

1. Skin rash, dermatitis, photosensitivity
2. Retinopathy
3. Muscular degeneration
4. Hypotension by IV use of chloroquine

Uses

1. In malaria
2. Hepatic amoebiasis
3. Giardiasis
4. Taeniasis
5. Rheumatoid arthritis
6. To control lepra reactions

Preparation

Chloroquine phosphate tablet IP.

Dose: 1 gm followed by 0.5 gm after 6 hours.

Brand Names

Resochin, Nivaquin, M-quin.

Q 3. Give the use, dose, route and brand names of following anti-malarial agents.

Drug	*Brand name*	*Use*	*Dose*	*Route*
Primaquine	Leoprime of malaria	Prophylaxis and treatment 14 days	15 mg daily for	Oral
Pyrimethamine	Daraprim cure of malaria	Prophylaxis and suppressive	25 mg weekly	Oral
Proguanil	Progunal	Prophylaxis of malaria	250 mg daily	Oral
Mepacrine	Mepalex of malaria	Prophylaxis and treatment daily for 5–7 days	100 mg thrice	

Q 4. Give the schematic representation of "life cycle of malarial parasites."

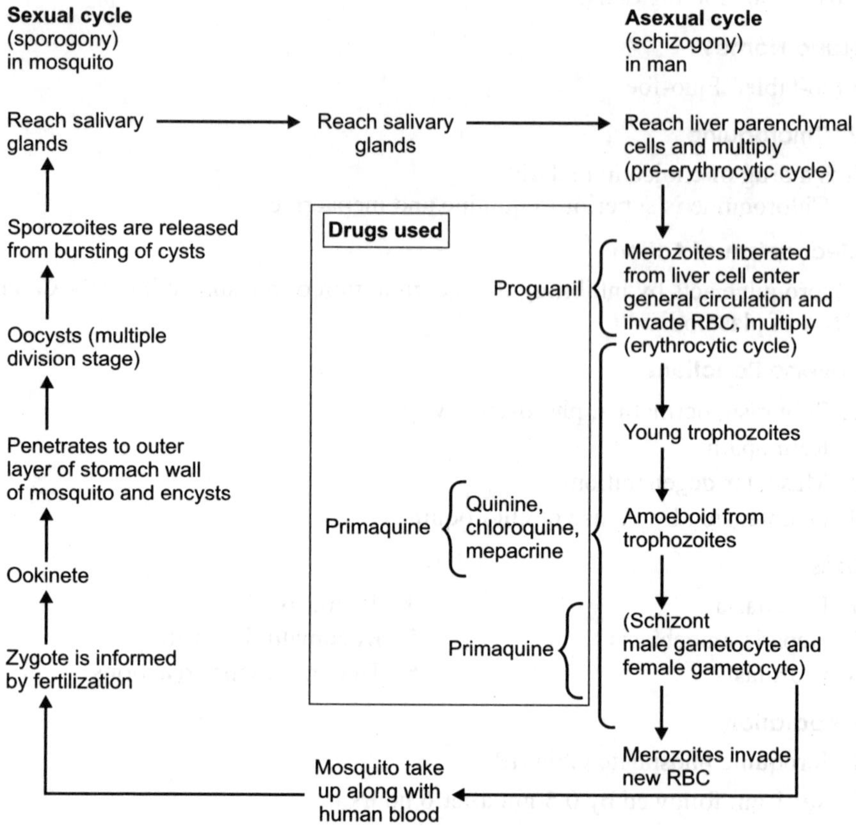

Schematic representation of "Life cycle of malarial parasite"

N. ANTINEOPLASTIC AGENTS

Q 1. Define and classify antineoplastic agents with examples.

Antineoplastic/Anticancer/Antitumour/Antimalignant/Cytotoxic Agents

The drugs which are used in the treatment of cancer are called antineoplastic agents/anticancer agents.

Classification

1. Alkylating agents:

a. *Nitrogen mustards:* Mechlorethamine, cyclophosphamide, melphalan, mustard, chlorambucil.

b. *Ethyleneimines:* Triethylenemelamine (TEM), triethylene thiophosphoramide (Thio TEPA).
c. *Alkyl sulfonates:* Busulfan.

2. **Antimetabolites:**
   a. Folic acid antagonist: Methotrexate.
   b. Purine antagonists: 6-mercaptopurine, azathioprine.
   c. Pyrimidine antagonists: Fluorouracil, cytosine arabinoside.
3. **Radioactive isotopes:** Radioiodine, radiophosphorus, radiogold.
4. **Antibiotics:** Actinomycin-D, rubidomycin, mitomycin, bleomycin.
5. **Hormones:** Androgens, estrogens, progestins, corticosteroid.
6. **Enzymes:** L-asparaginase.
7. **Miscellaneous agents:**
   a. Vinca alkaloids: Vincristine, vinblastine, taxol.
   b. Others: Hydroxyurea, cisplatin.

Q 2. Describe "alkylating agents used an antineoplastic agent."

Alkylating Agents

- These drugs act by the mechanism of alkylation, where the cell is negatively charged and combined with the agents positive components. This results in loss of cell proliferation and death. The action resembles to that produced by irradiation by ionising radiation, hence known as "radiomimetic substances."
- Alkylating agents were the first anticancer drugs used.
- Alkylating agents interfere with DNA replication by cross-linking DNA strands, DNA strand breaking and abnormal pairing of base pairs.
- The alkyl group is attached to the guanine base of DNA, at the number 7 nitrogen atom of the purine ring.
- Examples of alkylating agents:
  a. Cyclophosphamide
  b. Chlorambucil
  c. Busulphan
  d. Melphalan
  e. Triethylenemelamine (TEM)
  f. Thiotepa

a. Cyclophosphamide

- Cyclophosphamide is an alkylating agent used as anticancer agent.

Adverse Effects

- Nausea, vomiting, diarrhoea
- Hair loss
- Loss of appetite or weight
- Sores on mouth and tongue
- Changes in skin colour

Therapeutic uses

Cyclophosphamide is an anticancer, drug used to treat:

- Breast cancer
- Lung cancer
- Cancer of ovary
- Malignant lymphomas
- Chronic leukaemias
- Hodgkin's disease
- Neuroblastoma
- Ewing's sarcoma
- It is used as an immunosuppressive agent

Dosage

Cyclophosphamide injection IP.

Dose: 40–50 mg/kg in divided doses by IV

Brand Names

Cycloxan, Cytoxan, Endoxan.

b. Busulphan

- It is an alkylating agent used as antineoplastic.

Adverse Effects

- Aplasia of bone marrow
- Nausea, vomiting, diarrhoea, headache
- Constipation
- Dryness of mouth
- Loss of appetite or weight

Therapeutic uses

1. It is a cytotoxic agent
2. It is used to treat
   i. Chronic granulocytic leukaemia
   ii. Chronic myeloid leukaemia
3. In myelosclerosis
4. In polycythemia vera
5. In essential thrombocytopenia

Dosage

Busulphan tablet IP.

Dose: 2–4 mg daily orally.

Brand Names

Muleran, Misulban.

c. Chlorambucil

It is an alkylating agent used as antineoplastic agent.

Adverse Effects

- Nausea, vomiting
- Tiredness
- Missed menstrual periods
- Sources in mouth and throat

Therapeutic uses

1. It is useful in leukaemia and carcinoma of ovaries and testes.
2. To treat lymphocytic leukaemia.
3. To treat Hodgkin's disease.

Dosage

Chlorambucil tablet.

Dose: 0.1–0.2 mg/kg orally daily for 3–6 weeks as required.

Brand Name

Leukeran.

Q 3. What are antimetabolites? Explain the role of antimetabolites as antineoplastic agents.

Antimetabolites

- Antimetabolites are the substances with structural similarity with natural cell metabolites.
- They competitively inhibit the cell metabolite resulting into interference in cell growth.

  The antimetabolites useful as antineoplastic are:

  i. Purine analogues, e.g. 6-mercaptopurine.
  ii. Folic acid antagonist, methotrexate.
  iii. Pyrimidine antagonist, e.g. fluorouracil.
  iv. Glutamine antagonist, e.g. azaserine.

1. 6-mercaptopurine

- It is a purine analogue used as anticancer.
- It interferes with the synthesis of nucleic acid in the cell.
- It is useful in acute leukaemia.

Adverse Effects

- Leucopenia
- Thrombocytopenia
- Anorexia
- Vomiting and diarrhoea

Dosage

6-mercaptopurine tablet.

Dose: 2.5 mg/kg body weight daily, orally.

Brand Name

Purinethal.

2. Methotrexate

- Methotrexate is folic acid antagonist used as anticancer drug.
- Folic acid is natural metabolite in the cells. It is converted into dihydrofolic acid then into tetrahydrofolic acid which is useful in DNA synthesis the dihydrofolate reductase enzyme is responsible for further reaction is inhibited by methotrexate. Thus, resulting in cessation of DNA and RNA synthesis and shown antineoplastic action.

Adverse Effects

- Leucopenia
- Intestinal ulceration
- Thrombocytopenia
- Alopecia

Dosage

Methotrexate tablet.
Dose: 2.5–5 mg daily orally.

Brand Names

Reditrex, Trexall.

3. Fluorouracil

Fluorouracil is a pyrimidine antagonist used as anticancer agent.

Adverse Effects

- Nausea, headache
- Hair loss
- Dry and cracked skin
- Vision changes
- Dizziness

Therapeutic uses

1. It is a cytotoxic agent.
2. It is amost active drug against colorectal.
3. It is used to treat solar keratoses and other malignant conditions of skin.
4. It is used in the treatment of cancers of breast, colon, stomach, head, neck, bladder, etc.
5. Used in the palliative treatment of neoplasm of gastrointestinal tract, breast and pancreas and respiratory tract.

Dosage

Fluorouracil injection.
Dose: 12 mg/kg by IV once daily for 4 successive days.

Brand Name

Adrucil.

Objective Questions with Answers in Bold Letters

1. Diloxanide furoate is **antiamoebic agent**.
2. Metronidazole is a drug of choice in **amoebiasis**.
3. Malaria is caused by parasitic protozoa of genus **Plasmodium**.
4. Quinine is **schizonticidal**.
5. **Retinopathy** is major toxic effect of chloroquine.
6. **Cinchonism and black water fever** are the adverse effects of quinine.
7. The drugs used in the treatment of worms are called **anthelmintics**.
8. **Vermifuges** are the drugs which expel the worms from the body.
9. DEC stands for **diethyl carbamazine**.
10. Anthelmintics are administered with **purgatives**.
11. **Cyclophosphamide and chlorambucil** are alkylating agents used as antineoplastic drugs.
12. **Actinomycin-D** is an antibiotic used in treatment of cancer.
13. Vinblastine and vincristine are alkaloids used in treatment of **cancer**.
14. Alkylating agents are also called **"radiomimetic substance."**
15. Methotrexate is a **folic acid antagonist**.

Chapter 13

Biologicals

Q 1. What are biologicals? Give the sources and types of biologicals.

Biologicals

Biologicals are the medicines which are derived by using large scale cell cultures of bacteria, yeast, plants or animals.

- Biologicals are also known as biological therapeutics or biologics or biopharmaceuticals.
- Biologicals are used for prevention or treatment of diseases.
- Biologicals may be produced through biotechnology in living system.

Types

1. Immunotherapy: Cytokines, cancer treatment, vaccines, antibody.
2. Targeted therapies:
   i. Biological response modifier therapy (BRM therapy)
   ii. Biotherapy.
3. Blood components, blood derivatives, whole blood.
4. Proteins, xenotransplantation products.
5. Cellular and gene therapies.
6. Allergenic extracts.

Sources

1. Mammalian cell culture
2. Insect cell culture
3. Plant cell culture
4. Avian cell culture
5. Bacteria
6. Yeast
7. Transgenics
8. Humans

Q 2. Give the difference between biologicals and other drugs.

Biologicals	*Other drugs*
1. The large, complex, high molecular weight substances	1. These are small molecules
2. These are derived through biotechnology in living system	2. These are either synthesized in laboratories or extracted and purified from plants
3. As they stimulate immune responses, have safety concerns	3. Comparatively less safety concerns
4. They are complex, unique, large mixtures, not readily identifiable	4. They have well known chemical structure
5. They are very sensitive to heat	5. Majority of them are not sensitive to heat
6. Require aseptic conditions from initial manufacturing up to administration	6. May not require such conditions
7. They are administered by parenteral routes	7. Can be administered by different routes
8. They are costly	8. Not much costly
9. They are developed for rare, difficult to treat, disease states with no treatment options	9. They are useful for majority of disease conditions

Q 3. Give the indications/uses of biologicals (biologics).

Indications/uses of Biologicals (Biologics)

Biologicals are used/indicated in the following conditions:

- In rheumatoid arthritis
- In ankylosing spondylitis
- In psoriasis
- In Crohn's disease
- In ulcerative colitis
- In diabetes
- In multiple sclerosis
- In cervical cancer
- In hepatocellular cancer
- In chronic leukaemia

Examples of Biologicals and their uses

Rituximab: Non-Hodgkin's lymphoma, chronic lymphocytic leukaemia, rheumatoid arthritis, pemphigus vulgaris.

Avonex (interferon beta-1a): Multiple sclerosis.

Herceptin (trastuzumab): HER2-positive breast cancer, metastatic gastric and gastrooesophagal junction, adenocarcinoma.

Enbrel (etanercept): Rheumatoid arthritis, plaque psoriasis, psoriatic arthritis, ankylosing spondylitis.

Neulasta (pegfilgrastim): Neutropenia related to cancer chemotherapy.

Remicade (infliximab): Rheumatic arthritis, Crohn's disease, psoriatic arthritis, plaque psoriasis, ulcerative colitis.

Humira (adalimumab): It is one of the best selling drugs world wide used in rheumatoid arthritis, plaque psoriasis, Crohn's disease, ulcerative colitis.

Q. 4. Give the side effects of biologicals. Mention examples of biologicals.

Side Effects of Biolgicals

1. Most biologicals produce allergic hypersensitivity reactions.
2. Biologics used in rheumatic arthritis, and other immune-related disorders suppress the immune system and increase risk of infection.
3. Most biologics are given by injection and may cause injection site reactions.
4. Those given by IV infusion show infusion reactions.
5. Other side effects include chills, weakness, diarrhoea, nausea, rash, itching, shortness of breath, headache, fever, insomnia.

Examples/Biological Medicines

- Vaccines
- Blood and blood products
- Allergenics
- Somatic cells
- Gene therapy
- Recombinant therapy
- Hormones
- Cytokines
- Growth factors
- Insulin
- Interferon
- Monoclonal antibodies

Miscellaneous
(Objective Questions)

A. Antidotes used in Poisoning Cases

1. Morpine poisoning: Naloxone, nalorphine.
   (opium poisoning)
2. Atropine poisoning (belladonna poisoning): Physostigmine.
3. Organophosphorus poisoning: Atropine, pralidoxime.
4. Nicotine poisoning: Clonidine, haloperidol.
5. Strychnine poisoning: Diazepam, barbiturates.
6. Digitalis poisoning: Potassium chloride.
7. Alcohol poisoning: Disulfiram.
8. Salicylate poisoning: Sodium bicarbonate.
9. Barbiturate poisoning: Sodium thiosulphate, sodium nitrite.
10. Cyanide poisoning: Sodium thiosulphate, sodium nitrite.
11. Insecticide poisoning: Atropine.
12. Carbon monoxide poisoning: Oxygen.
13. Bromide poisoning: Sodium chloride.
14. Mercury, gold, arsenic poisoning: Dimercaprol (BAL).
15. Lead, copper, manganese poisoning: Calcium disodium edetate.
16. Copper, mercury: Penicillamine.
17. Iron poisoning: Desferrioxamine.

B. Inhibitors and Blockers

1. β-Blockers: Ergotamine, phentolamine, tolazoline, phenoxybenzamine.
2. β-Blockers: Propranolol, labetalol, atenolol, metoprolol.
3. Adrenergic neuron blockers: Guanethidine, reserpine.
4. Neuromuscular blockers: Gallamine, succinylcholine, d-tubocurarine.
5. Ganglionic blockers: Mecamylamine, hexamethonium.
6. Calcium channel blockers: Verapamil, nifedipine.
7. MAO inhibitors: Isocarboxazid, phenelzine, pargyline.
8. Cholinesterase inhibitors: Physostigmine, neostigmine, pyridostigmine.
9. Carbonic anhydrase inhibitors: Acetazolamide, methazolamide.

10. ACE inhibitors (angiotensin converting enzyme inhibitors): Captopril, enalapril.
11. Na^+, K^+ ATPase inhibitor: Digitalis (digoxin).
12. Prostaglandin synthesis inhibitor: Aspirin.

C. Major Adverse/Toxic Effects

1. Gray baby syndrome: Chloramphenicol.
2. Ototoxicity: Streptomycin.
3. Discolouration of teeth: Tetracycline
4. Allergy (anaphylaxis): Penicillin
5. Triple response: Histamine
6. Constipation: Morphine, atropine
7. Black water fever: Quinine
8. Retinopathy: Chloroquine
9. Metallic taste in mouth: Metronidazole
10. Dryness of mouth: Atropine
11. Methaemoglobinemia: Dapsone
12. Liver toxicity: Chloroform
13. Photophobia: Atropine
14. Peripheral neuritis: Isoniazid
15. Drug automatism: Phenobarbitone
16. Urinary retention: Atropine, morphine
17. Cyanosis: Chloramphenicol
18. Suicidal tendencies: Diazepam, morphine
19. Palpitation: Adrenaline, ephedrine
20. Cinchonism: Quinine
21. Pin-point pupil: Morphine
22. Haematuria: Dapsone
23. Bone marrow depression: Chloramphenicol
24. Hypokalemia: Chlorthiazide, digitalis
25. Parkinsonism: Chlorpromazine, methyldopa
26. Anorexia: Amphetamine, carbamazepine
27. Parasthesia: Physostigmine, neostigmine
28. Cholestatic jaundice: Imipramine
29. Difficulty in micturition: Atropine
30. Nephrotoxicity: Cephalosporins
31. Aplastic anemia: Chloramphenicol
32. Obstruction in urine flow: Sulphonamides
33. Cardiac arrest: Acetylcholine

34. Damage to vestibulocochlear nerve (auditory/8th cranial/ deafness): Streptomycin.
35. Difficulty in swallowing: Atropine
36. Agranulocytosis: Chloramphenicol
37. Pin-point pupil: Morphine
38. Blurring of vision: Chloroquine
39. Postural hypotension: Methyldopa
40. Obstructive jaundice: Erythromycin
41. Blood dyscrasia: Paracetamol
42. Heartburn: Aspirin
43. Haemorrhage: Warfarin
44. Peptic ulceration: Aspirin
45. Euphoria: Morphine, heroin
46. Diplopia: Atropine, primidone
47. Mental clouding: Morphine, lignocaine
48. Cycloplegia/dysphagia: Atropine
49. Tremors: Adrenaline, ephedrine
50. Thrombocytopenia: Quinidine
51. Rebound hypertension: Methyldopa
52. Hyperkalemia: Spironolactone
53. Alopecia: Heparin
54. Hypoglycemia: Insulin
55. Rebound acidity: Sodium bicarbonate
56. Stevens-Johnson syndrome: Sulphadiazine, sulphadimidine
57. Crystalluria: Sulphonamides
58. Presbiopia: Insulin
59. Glossitis: Penicillin-G
60. Colitis: Amoxycillin, ampicillin
61. Eosinophilia: Erythromycin
62. Hypoplasia of gums: Tetracycline

D. Mention the Drugs of Choice

1. Peptic ulcer: Cimetidine, ranitidine
2. Status epilepticus: Diazepam
3. Myasthenia gravis: Neostigmine
4. Status asthmaticus: Hydrocortisone
5. Parkinsonism: Levodopa, carbidopa
6. Bronchial asthma: Adrenaline
7. Grand mal epilepsy: Phenytoin
8. Constipation: Castor oil, senna

9. Diarrhoea: Loperamide, atropine
10. Glaucoma: Pilocarpine
11. Motion sickness: Promethazine
12. Angina pectoris: Glyceryl trinitrate
13. Thyrotoxicosis: Carbimazole, methimazole
14. Gout: Colchicine, probenecid
15. Rheumatism: Indomethacin, aspirin
16. Obesity: Amphetamine
17. Cycloplegia: Pilocarpine
18. Schizophrenia: Chlorpromazine
19. Depression: Imipramine
20. Heart block: Adrenaline, isoprenaline
21. CCF/CHF: Digitalis
22. Migraine: Aspirin
23. Diabetes mellitus: Insulin
24. Tonsillitis: Cotrimoxazole
25. Stokes-Adams syndrome: Adrenaline
26. Narcolepsy: Ephedrine, amphetamine
27. Insomnia: Diazepam, phenobarbitone
28. Raynaud's disease: Tolazoline
29. Oedema: Frusemide, mannitol
30. Paralytic ileus: Carbachol, bethanechol
31. Dropsy: Frusemide
32. Hypertension: Clonidine, methyldopa
33. Anxiety: Diazepam, nitrazepam
34. Eosinophilia: Iron, vitamin B_{12}
35. Pellagra: Nikethamide
36. Spondylitis: Phenylbutazone
37. Psychosis: Chlorpromazine
38. Haemorrhage: Thrombin, menadione
39. Bradycardia: Isoprenaline
40. Tachycardia: Propranolol, digoxin
41. Thrombosis: Heparin
42. Diabetes insipidus: Vasopressin
43. Hyperthyroidism: Propylthiouracil
44. Whooping cough: Ephedrine
45. Amoebiasis: Metronidazole
46. Helminthiasis: Piperazine
47. Candidiasis: Nystatin, griseofulvin

48. Ascariasis: Piperazine, tetramisole
49. Oxyuriasis: Pyrantel pamoate
50. Giardiasis: Metronidazole
51. Onychomycosis: Griseofulvin, nystatin
52. Blastomycosis: Amphotericin
53. Trichomoniasis: Metronidazole
54. Plague: Tetracycline
55. Typhoid and paratyphoid: Chloramphenicol
56. Meningitis: Benzylpenicillin
57. Tuberculosis: Isoniazid, ethambutol
58. Leprosy: Dapsone, solapsone
59. Malaria: Quinine, chloroquine
60. Hookworm infestation: Albendazole
61. Malignancy: Busulphan, chlorambucil
62. Trachoma: Chloramphenicol
63. Gonorrhoea: Penicillin-G
64. Urinary tract infection: Streptomycin
65. Rheumatic fever: Penicillin-G
66. Embolism: Heparin
67. Lumbago, sciatica: Aspirin, paracetamol
68. Mania: Imipramine
69. Pheochromocytoma: Propranolol
70. Arteriosclerosis: Clofibrate, nicotinic acid.

E. Name one drug each contraindicated in the following conditions

1. Glaucoma: Atropine
2. Prostate enlargement: Propranolol, testosterone
3. Peptic ulcer: Aspirin, reserpine
4. Cirrhosis of liver: Phenobarbitone, alcohol
5. Impairment of renal function: Sulfa drugs
6. Hypertension: Adrenaline
7. Congestive cardiac failure: Quinidine
8. Bronchial asthma: Acetylcholine, carbachol
9. Stokes-Adams syndrome: Quinidine
10. Intestinal obstruction: Atropine, morphine
11. Head injury: Morphine (brain injury)
12. Insomnia: Bemegride, nikethamide
13. Pheochromocytoma: Methyldopa, guanethidine
14. Myasthenia gravis: Streptomycin, kanamycin.

Pharmacology

Sample Question Paper 1
(As Per PCI Format)

Time: 03 Hours | Marks: 80

Q 1. Attempt any *six* of the following: (5 × 6 = 30 Marks)

a. Classify routes of administration of drugs. Give advantages and disadvantages of oral route.

b. Define and classify anticholinergic. Explain in detail atropine.

c. What is preanaesthetic medication? Give the reasons and drugs used in preanaesthetic medication. Describe in brief basal anaesthesia.

d. Define cardiotonics. Describe the drugs used in congestive heart failure.

e. What are antibiotics? Write a note on penicillins.

f. What is cotrimoxazole? Give its mechanism of action, uses, adverse effects, dosage, and brand names.

g. Give the reasons:

  i. Why acetazolamide is a self-limiting diuretics?

  ii. Why adrenaline is always present as an emergency kit of the physician?

Q 2. Attempt any *ten* of the following: (3 × 10 = 30 Marks)

a. Describe oral hypoglycemic agents.

b. Write a note on "acute barbiturate poisoning".

c. What is hypertension? Define and classify antihypertensive agents giving examples.

d. Write note on drugs used in: i. Glaucoma; ii. Status asthmaticus.

e. What are autocoids? Explain triple response.

f. Mention the drugs contraindicated in the following conditions:

  i. Pregnancy

  ii. Glaucoma

  iii. Cirohosis of liver

  iv. Pheochromocytoma

  v. Hypertension

  vi. Prostate enlargement

g. Define and classify antineoplastic drugs with examples.

h. Define biologicals. Give the indications/uses of biologicals.
i. What are aminoglycoside antibiotics? Give examples.
j. Write in brief pharmacology of: i. Calcitonin; ii. Oxytocin.
k. Name one drug each producing one of the following toxic effects:
   i. Hepatotoxicity
   ii. Ototoxicity
   iii. Allergy
   iv. Constipation
   v. Alopecia
   vi. Peptic ulcer

Q 3. Attempt *all* questions of the following: (1 × 20 = 20 Marks)

a. Glyceryl trinitrate in the treatment of angina pectoris is given by:
   i. SC route
   ii. Rectal route
   iii. IV route
   iv. Sublingual route
b. Which of the following is not a process of absorption of drug?
   i. Passive diffusion
   ii. Active transport
   iii. Pinocytosis
   iv. Cumulation
c. Which of the following gas is known as "laughing gas"?
   i. Oxygen
   ii. Sulphur dioxide
   iii. Nitrous oxide
   iv. Carbon dioxide
d. Name the antidote used in organophosphorus poisoning.
e. Long form of NSAIDs is _______________.
f. Give two examples of β-blockers.
g. _______________ is a branch of science deals with study of doses of drugs.
h. Enemas are administered by which route?
i. Name the toxicity having harmful effects of drugs on foetus.
j. The person fails to respond to bright light is known as ____________.
k. Which vitamin is called cholecalciferol?
l. IDDM stands for _______________.
m. Dale's vasomotor reversal phenomenon is produced by which drug?
n. State one drug used in treatment of atherosclerosis.
o. Give one example of drug used as antiamoebic.
p. Name the drug whose popular brand name is "Largactil".
q. 'Dulcolax' is a popular brand name of which drug?
r. What is the source of heparin?
s. Name of the antidote used in acute salicylate poisoning.
t. Define mydriatics.

Pharmacology

Sample Question Paper 2
(As Per PCI Format)

Time: 03 Hours | Marks: 80

Q 1. Attempt any *six* of the following: (5 × 6 = 30 Marks)

a. What is epilepsy? Explain types of epilepsy. Classify anticonvulsant drugs giving suitable examples.

b. Define and classify diuretics. Give the indications of diuretics.

c. Write a note on drugs used in angina pectoris.

d. What is bronchial asthma? Give the different forms of bronchial asthma and its treatment. Write in brief about treatment of status asthmaticus.

e. Describe thrombolytic agents.

f. Define nootropic. Explain various nootropic agents.

g. Give reasons:

   i. Why the drugs are given in combination in the treatment of tuberculosis?

   ii. Why eating of cheese is forbidden in patients with MAO inhibitor therapy?

Q 2. Attempt any *ten* of the following: (3 × 10 = 30 Marks)

a. What is parenteral route? Give merits and demerits of parenteral route.

b. Define and classify local anaesthetics. Give the properties of an ideal local anaesthetic drugs.

c. Define antagonism. Explain types of antagonism.

d. Describe antiulcer drugs that reduce gastric acid secretions.

e. Explain Dale's vasomotor reversal phenomenon.

f. Mention the drug of choice in the following conditions:

   i. Thyrotoxicosis
   ii. Gout
   iii. Plague
   iv. Myasthenia gravis
   v. Depression
   vi. Helminthiasis

g. Write a note on parathormone.

h. Explain “insulin as a hypoglycemic agent”. Give the preparations of insulin.

i. Write an account of progesterone.

j. What is tuberculosis? Define and classify antitubercular agent. Add a note on isoniazid.

k. Give brief an account of ‘drugs used in HIV infection’.

Q 3. Attempt *all* questions of the following: (1 × 20 = 20 Marks)

a. Which drug is called cardiotonic?

b. Define anthelminitics.

c. Give the long form of NIDDM ______________.

d. Mebendazole is used as ______________.

e. Enlist an example of carbonic anhydrase inhibitor.

f. Name the organism which causes amoebiasis.

g. INH stands for ______________.

h. Xylocaine is a popular brand name of which drugs?

i. Give one example of lipid lowering agent.

j. Nalorphine and naloxone are antidote used in which poisoning?

k. Give the use of castor oil.

l. Give two examples of H_2-antagonists.

m. What is dose of pralidoxime?

n. Name of the drug which produces muscarinic and nicotinic action.

o. Define bactericides.

p. Give the source of streptomycin.

q. Cinchonism and black water fever are the major toxic effects of which drug?

r. What is vermifuge?

s. Insomnia means ______________.

t. Insulin is used in the treatment of ______________.